D0907094

DISCARD

Smart Medicine

for a Healthy

Prostate

Smart Medicine for a Healthy Prostate

Natural and Conventional Therapies
for Common Prostate Disorders

Mark W. McClure, M.D.

Foreword by Robert S. Ivker, D.O.

Avery

a member of

Penguin Putnam Inc.

New York

Most Avery books are available at special quantity discounts for bulk purchase for sales promotions, premiums, fund-raising, and educational needs. Special books or book excerpts also can be created to fit specific needs. For details, write Putnam Special Markets, 375 Hudson Street, New York, NY 10014.

AVERY

a member of
Penguin Putnam Inc.
375 Hudson Street
New York, NY 10014
www.penguinputnam.com

Library of Congress Cataloging-in-Publication Data

McClure, Mark W.
Smart medicine for a healthy prostate : natural and conventional
therapies for common prostate disorders / Mark W. McClure.
p.   cm.
Includes bibliographical references and index.
ISBN 1-58333-113-1
1. Prostate—Diseases—Popular works.   I. Title.
RC899 .M396   2001   2001033665
616.6'5—dc21

Printed in the United States of America
1   3   5   7   9   10   8   6   4   2

Book design by Meighan Cavanaugh

I dedicate this book to Bobby Anderson,
and to all of my other patients who've shared
their healing journeys with me.

Acknowledgments

I wish to thank Rudy Shur for believing in me and giving me the opportunity to write this book. I am also indebted to my many mentors in conventional and complementary medicine. My patients deserve special thanks as well for sharing their healing stories with me, offering to read my manuscript, and sharing their insights. I also wish to acknowledge the librarian staff at Wake Medical Center for assisting me with my research; Jeff Hickman for his help and friendship; Drew Griffin and Fran Sapir for their expertise and encouragement; and Eric Yarnell, N.D., for his tutelage in herbal matters. Furthermore, I am especially indebted to Michael Lutfy, Dara Stewart, and the rest of the editorial staff at Avery Publishing Group and Penguin Putnam for guiding me through the various stages of my book's birthing process. Finally, I am humbled by the steadfast faith and support of my best friend and partner, Cheri Elliott, who took a chance on love, opened up her heart, and enthusiastically agreed to skip down the road of life with me.

Contents

*The doctor of the future
will give no medicine, but will interest his [her] patients
in the care of the human frame, nutrition, and the
cause and prevention of disease.*

THOMAS EDISON

Foreword

Smart Medicine for a Healthy Prostate could not have been written at a better time for men. Despite the advances in medical technology and research, statistics show that American men, to a much greater extent than American women, have experienced a steady decline in both physical and emotional health:

- Life expectancy for men is seven years shorter than it is for women.
- Prostate cancer afflicts one out of nine men and kills about 40,000 of them each year. In the last five years, the death rate for this most common cancer in men has grown almost twice as fast as that of breast cancer.
- 80 percent of all suicides and serious drug addicts are men.
- Men are three times as likely as women to be alcoholics and are 25 times as likely to end up in prison.

Part of the problem is that men have been mentally conditioned with attitudes that have taught us that "if it ain't broke, don't fix it," "big boys don't cry," "it's not cool to be fearful," and that it's admirable to "play with pain and suck it up." Possibly most damaging to us is the belief that the formula for success and happiness is an abundance of money, power, winning, and sex. This unhealthy thinking, combined with a frighteningly low level of emotional intelligence, a fear of intimacy, and a lack of meaning and purpose, has taken a huge toll on our prostates, our hearts (heart disease is the leading killer of men), and the rest of our bodies, while also leading to multiple addictions. Even though these mental/emotional and spiritual/social factors play enormous roles in creating physical "dis-ease," there are other important factors as well, such as heredity, poor diet, daily exposure to a multitude of environmental toxins, and lack of adequate exercise. But be aware that it is not simply genetics that causes half of all men over 60 to develop enlarged prostates, one in five men over 70 to develop prostate cancer, two million men to visit doctors for prostatitis each year, and an astounding 30 million men to become impotent!

To experience optimal health and not simply prostate health, men have to transcend their quest to "fix the broken part." They must become more conscious of how to care for themselves: learn what makes them feel better both physically and emotionally, identify the factors that make them feel worse and weaken their prostates, and learn how to prevent prostate disease. This book is an excellent manual to help guide men in this exhilarating healing process.

I have never seen a more comprehensive self-help book on prostate health in my 30 years as a family physician. Dr. McClure is a healer, a holistic urologist, and a medical pioneer who has helped to establish holistic medicine as American medicine's newest specialty. This book provides a wide array of effective options to help men love and nurture their prostates as they treat and prevent prostate dysfunction and heal their lives. But to fully benefit from the therapies and wisdom that Mark McClure is offering you on the following pages requires *a commitment to changing your life.* And while you're focusing on your prostate, you'll be restoring balance and harmony to the rest of your body and to your mind and spirit. The extent to which you follow his recommendations—especially the complementary therapies—for treating, preventing, and possibly curing prostate cancer, prostatitis, and prostate enlargement will have a high degree of correlation to your levels of energy and vitality and to your peace of mind, self-acceptance, self-esteem, and intimacy with your wife, partner, and God.

Smart Medicine presents an art and science that holistic physicians regard as the ultimate form of preventive medicine. It will enable you to heighten your self-awareness and will empower you to take charge of your life. What do you have to lose? I wish you well on your journey!

Robert S. Ivker, D.O., is the past president of the American Holistic Medical Association and author of the best-selling books *Sinus Survival* and *The Self-Care Guide to Holistic Medicine.*

Smart Medicine

for a Healthy

Prostate

Introduction

If you have picked up this book, then the chances are good that you or someone you know has one of the three prostate conditions that is discussed in the pages that follow. You are not alone. At one time or another, most men will be affected by at least one of these prostate problems. To put matters in perspective, prostate cancer—the leading cause of cancer in men—can begin as early as puberty and affects nearly every man if he lives long enough. Prostate enlargement, another common condition, affects half of all men over the age of sixty, one-third of whom need treatment. Finally, prostatitis accounts for more than two million doctor visits yearly. In fact, prostatitis is the most frequent reason that men under the age of fifty see a urologist.

That's the bad news—now for the good news. You don't have to become one of these statistics. If you're blessed with a healthy prostate, I'll show you how to keep it that way. If you're afflicted with prostate disease, I'll show you how to overcome it. Either way, *Smart Medicine for a Healthy Prostate* is intended for men of all ages. Based on information I've gathered from scientific research, coupled with more than twenty years of professional experience as a physician, urologic surgeon, and practitioner of conventional and complementary medicine, my book will help you achieve optimal prostate health.

Complementary vs. Conventional Medicine

Before we get to the subject of prostate health, however, I think it is necessary to define what complementary medicine is and how it differs from conventional medicine and alternative medicine. In recent years, the integration of alternative medicine with conventional medicine has become popularly known as complementary medicine. The term *alternative medicine* refers to any treatment or healing system that is not considered "mainstream" by the accepted medical establishment. For example, organized medicine classifies herbal therapies as alternative medicine. In many other parts of the world, the situation is reversed. Herbal therapies are "mainstream" medicine for more than 80 percent of the world's population, while expensive prescription drugs and surgery are regarded as alternative medicine. For the purposes of this book, the alternative therapies that are used to complement conventional therapies for prostate disease include diet, lifestyle, vitamins, supplements, herbal medicine, mind-body medicine, and various forms of behavioral medicine.

As a urologist who practices both conventional and complementary medicine, I wear two hats. When I don my conventional medicine hat, I'm able to offer patients state-of-the-art therapies, the best that modern science has to offer. But by donning my other hat, I'm able to offer men complementary therapies that make conventional therapies more effective. In addition, complementary therapies cost less, have fewer side effects, and frequently work when conventional remedies have failed.

Unfortunately, my medical colleagues often advise their patients not to use alternative therapies, claiming that these therapies lack scientific support. In spite of these claims, a growing body of scientific evidence suggests otherwise. In the following chapters, I present a wide assortment of "evidence-based" alternative therapies for prostate disease. (Evidence-based therapies have been subjected to scientific research and found to be effective.) The results of these data have been published in peer-reviewed journals—professional journals that accept only articles that meet agreed-upon standards.

Complementary medicine and conventional medicine each has its strengths and weaknesses. For instance, conventional medicine excels at handling medical emergencies such as trauma, heart attacks, acute bacterial infection, and reconstructive surgery. However, conventional medicine can be less effective for treating chronic illnesses such as diabetes, heart disease, cancer, and mental illness.

By contrast, complementary medicine is not well suited to handle acute medical emergencies, but it does a much better job of treating chronic illness. For example, conventional drug therapies help only a third of the men with nonbacterial chronic prostatitis—an ill-defined, noninfectious prostate disease that plagues millions of men. Complementary therapies (such as muscle relaxation, stress reduction, and selected nutritional supplements) help the majority of these men.

BASIC PHILOSOPHICAL DIFFERENCES

The main difference in the success rate between these two therapies can be traced to the fact that conventional medicine focuses on treating the *disease,* whereas complementary medicine focuses on treating the *patient.*

Practitioners of conventional medicine believe that a malfunction of the body can always be explained by a particular abnormality that is caused on a biological, cellular, tissue, or organ level. By contrast, complementary medicine views *dis-ease,* meaning "not at ease," as an imbalance within the body that stems from a breakdown in the weblike interaction among mind, body, spirit, and environment. Because this imbalance is unique to the individual, so should be the treatment.

Finally, in complementary medicine, dis-ease is differentiated from illness. Dis-ease is the underlying imbalance that causes symptoms. Although related to dis-ease, illness is what patients experience on a physical, psychological, and spiritual level because of their disease.

DIAGNOSIS

Complementary medicine and conventional medicine also differ in their approach to diagnosis. Although practitioners of both evaluate a patient's signs (physical findings) and symptoms (complaints) to reach a diagnosis, their perspective techniques are quite different.

In conventional medicine, diagnosis is defined as the art of distinguishing one disease from another or discovering the nature of a disease. The results of "hard data" (laboratory and high-tech tests) are given greater weight than those of "soft data" (intuition and the patients narra-

tive of illness). By a process of elimination, doctors arrive at a "working diagnosis" (educated guess) that they use to name a patient's complaints. In
conventional medicine, subsequent treatments are based on the disease's
name.

In this era of technological wizardry, it may seem an anachronism to
some that careful listening is the diagnostic test most valued by practitioners of complementary medicine. Valuable clues gleaned from attentive
history taking are unobtainable by any other means, including the most
sophisticated testing.

THERAPEUTIC APPROACH

Based on the assigned diagnosis (name of the disease), doctors of conventional medicine treat illness with external means, usually by dispensing
drugs or performing surgery. In conventional medicine, the patient plays
a passive role: The medical doctor dictates a treatment that the patient is
expected to follow.

However, the goal of complementary medicine is not to treat disease
but to correct the imbalance in the body by restoring its natural healing capacity. To facilitate this process, doctors who practice complementary medicine begin by educating their patients. Patients are taught how to access the
skills and resources they need for self-healing. They are expected to take an
active role in their healing process. They're also invited to explore the
deeper meaning of their illness. Doctors literally formulate a treatment plan
that is coauthored with their patients. When complementary therapies are
called for, the minimal therapy that will restore balance is used.

Finally, doctors who practice complementary medicine realize that
health is more than the absence of disease. Therefore, they help their patients to devise a program of preventive health that they can use to achieve
optimal health.

RISKS OF SELF-DIAGNOSIS

Whereas many physicians are unaware of the benefits that alternative and
complementary medicine have to offer, their patients are not. In fact, sta-

tistics show that more than 40 percent of Americans use alternative medicine. Unfortunately, though, not all alternative therapies are created equal—some work, others don't, and some can cause harm. Furthermore, treating symptoms (complaints) without first knowing the cause can be risky business.

For instance, three typical symptoms of prostate disease are difficult, frequent, and urgent urination. While these symptoms are usually caused by benign (noncancerous) conditions such as prostate enlargement or prostatitis, a more serious condition such as prostate cancer can cause identical symptoms. On the one hand, prostate cancer is best managed with a combination of conventional and complementary therapies. On the other hand, prostate enlargement and prostatitis can often be safely treated with complementary therapies alone. The only way to differentiate among these three conditions, though, is a thorough medical evaluation. Therefore, since failure to make the right diagnosis can have dire consequences, I recommend seeking professional medical advice before embarking on a trial of complementary therapies.

Nutritional Supplements

Nutritional supplements, such as vitamins, minerals, amino acids, antioxidants, natural food–derived products, and herbs, are the essence of complementary medicine and are therefore mentioned throughout this book. You'll learn that these nutritional supplements can help prevent prostate disease, decrease side effects of conventional therapies, and improve the quality of life.

In general, I advise all of my patients to supplement their diet with a high-potency multivitamin and take selected nutritional supplements. At the same time, I remind them that taking vitamins and supplements won't prevent or counteract the damage that is caused by a combination of poor dietary habits, poor lifestyle choices, poor exercise routines, and a poor outlook on life.

Although an in-depth discussion of nutritional supplements is beyond the scope of this book, I've organized a brief overview of nutritional supplements and listed other valuable resources in the appendices. I strongly recommend that you explore these resources to complement the information in this book, and as part of your continuing education on maintaining your overall health.

How to Select a Physician

Now that you're committed to achieving optimal health and learning more about complementary medicine, how do you go about finding the right doctor? The following criteria will serve as a helpful guide.

Unfortunately, many patients have been dissuaded from exploring complementary medicine because of a disparaging remark that their doctor made about complementary medicine. Gut-level reactions to alternatives like herbs (instead of conventional treatments such as drugs and surgery) typically stem from prejudice that is taught in traditional medical school and residency training. Negative pronouncements of organized medical organizations, such as the American Medical Association, have also hampered honest inquiry.

But a good physician should be open-minded enough to consider which approach is in the best interest of his or her patient. If your physician scoffs at the very idea of using complementary medicine without first investigating the possible benefits, then perhaps you might want to look for another doctor.

Physicians best demonstrate their professionalism by how they treat their patients. HMOs and other factors have created a situation where doctors spend less time with their patients than ever before. There is a not-so-funny aphorism popular among doctors that says, "When all else fails, talk to the patient." Caring, professional doctors are those who:

- take the time to perform a thorough history and exam
- listen carefully to what patients have to say
- are willing to answer all of their questions
- are intellectually honest and willing to research a question they may not know the answer to

Finally, don't be afraid to ask your doctor about his or her training. For conventional medicine proficiency, I recommend selecting a physician who is board certified. A board-certified physician has successfully completed medical school and residency training in an accredited institution, then passed a series of written and oral proficiency examinations that are given by an accrediting specialty board.

Since the field of complementary medicine is relatively new, establishing a doctor's proficiency in complementary medicine is more challenging. You might start by asking how he or she became interested in complementary and alternative medicine; about any specialized training; and about his or her program of continuing medical education. Furthermore, if a doctor offers specialized procedures, such as acupuncture, ask if he or she is certified by an accredited specialty organization. Alternatively, you can call the appropriate accrediting agency yourself and find out if the physician is a member in good standing. In the year 2000, the American Board of Holistic Medicine began offering board certification in holistic medicine to qualified physicians. As a note of interest, I successfully completed the examination and became a founding member of the American Board of Holistic Medicine.

How to Use This Book

This book is organized into four chapters. In the first chapter, I offer a very basic overview of the prostate and pertinent male anatomy, which I strongly recommend you read first. It is essential that you have a thorough understanding of the prostate and its function before we discuss what can go wrong and possible treatment.

In each of the other three chapters, I cover a different prostate disease. Each chapter is organized in a similar fashion. In the first half of each chapter, I provide information about the natural history, evaluation, and conventional therapies for the condition. In the second half, I outline proven complementary therapies that are based on scientific research, and point out what you need to know and how to apply it.

Finally, in the last section of the book, you'll find appendices with information on supplements and a list of valuable resources.

1

An Overview of the Prostate and Its Function

Most men are blissfully unaware of their prostate gland because it's tucked out of sight, out of mind. But the prostate commands immediate attention if it develops plumbing problems. Situated right in the middle of the urinary and reproductive systems, the prostate can wreak havoc with both systems. But in the chapters that follow, I'll give you a preventive maintenance program as well as a repair guide for three of the most common prostate maladies. Before getting started, though, I highly recommend that you read the following prostate "owner's manual."

Prostate Overview

Before we cover the function of the prostate, let's go over some basic prostate anatomy. It is important that you have some understanding of all the parts involved so you can understand how they interact and what can go wrong.

BASIC PROSTATE ANATOMY

The prostate is situated in a strategic position, just outside the bladder, beneath the pubic bone, anterior (on the abdominal side) to the rectum

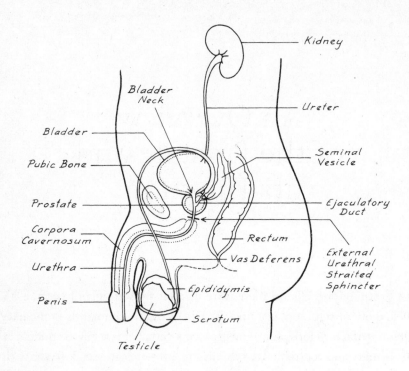

FIGURE 1.1 *Male Genitourinary Anatomy*

(see Figure 1.1 above). Fibrous attachments from the pubic bone above, and muscular attachments where the bladder joins the prostate and laterally on both sides, keep the prostate securely in place. (Since the prostate rests just outside the rectum, doctors can feel the outside surface of the prostate by doing a digital rectal examination. See Figure 4 on page 33.)

Bladder

The bladder is a hollow muscular organ that stores urine. At the *bladder neck,* where the bladder joins the prostate, muscle fibers from both organs interweave to form a sphincter muscle called the *internal sphincter.* Sphincter muscles control the passage of urine by either relaxing (opening) to allow urine to pass or contracting (closing) to prevent its passage. The internal sphincter is normally closed, except during urination.

Urethra

Urine is passed through a hollow tube about three-eighths of an inch in diameter called the *urethra*. The urethra originates where the prostate meets the bladder, continues through the middle of the prostate, and then extends the length of the penis.

Although the size varies, the *prostatic urethra*—the section of urethra that passes through the prostate itself—usually measures an inch or two in length. The inside where the urethra is in contact with urine is lined with *transitional cells,* the same type of cells that line the inside layer of the bladder. On the outside, the urethra is firmly attached to the surrounding prostate tissue. A series of *prostatic ducts* carrying fluid from the prostate, and a pair of *ejaculatory ducts* carrying fluid from the *vasa* (paired vas deferens) and *seminal vesicles,* enter the floor of the prostatic urethra on either side (more on this later).

To help you visualize the relationship of the urethra to the rest of the prostate, imagine the prostate as an apple, with the urethra as its core, only hollow, and the prostate tissue as its fruit. Surrounding the prostate, like apple skin, is a tough fibrous covering called the *prostatic capsule.* Since prostate tissue surrounds the urethra, people often wonder how prostate tissue can be removed without destroying the urethra in the process. Well, guess what? The urethra *is* destroyed, just as an apple core is destroyed when it's cored out, but, miraculous as it may seem, the raw surface of the remaining prostate tissue forms a healthy new urethral lining within a matter of weeks.

Muscle Contractions

A voluntary muscle called the *external urethral striated sphincter* surrounds the urethra just distal (away from) the prostate, opposite the bladder. Striated muscles, which have a "row-like" (striated) appearance under the microscope, are under conscious control; that is, they can be contracted and relaxed at will to stop or permit the flow of urine.

The Supply System

A network of nerves, arteries, veins, and lymphatic vessels supplies the prostate. Nerves relay messages to receptors that are located on smooth

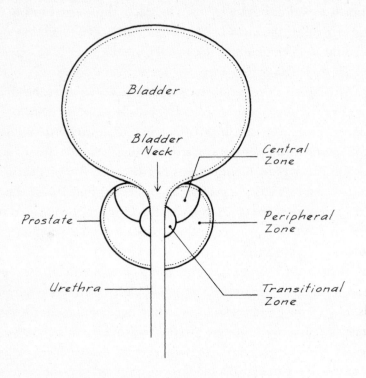

FIGURE 1.2 *The Zones of the Prostate*

muscle fibers in the prostate tissue, bladder neck, and prostatic capsule. Depending on the messages received, these muscle fibers either contract or relax. As you'll learn in the next chapter, conventional and natural therapies for prostate enlargement target nerves that constrict smooth muscle tissue, since increased smooth muscle tone causes prostatic obstruction. Arteries that supply the prostate deliver oxygen, nutrients, and immune cells throughout the prostate, and veins that accompany these arteries carry blood back to the heart. Lymphatic vessels drain waste material from the prostate and coalesce near blood vessels in the lower abdomen to form dime-sized filtration stations called lymph nodes. When the prostate is diseased, tumor cells and infected prostatic secretions can be transported to other parts of the body via the venous and lymphatic systems.

Similarly, if the prostate is inflamed, pain can be referred elsewhere via nerves that supply and surround the prostate.

Prostate Zones

According to scientific research, the prostate is composed of three zones: the *transitional zone,* which surrounds the urethra, accounts for 5 percent of the total prostate volume; the *central zone,* which lays adjacent to the transitional zone, accounts for 20 percent of the prostate volume; and the *peripheral zone,* which occupies the outer portion of the prostate, accounts for the remaining prostate volume (see Figure 1.2 on page 13). (Although useful for descriptive purposes, in real life there aren't clear-cut demarcations among the three zones.)

Prostate Tissue

Prostate tissue contains a complex mixture of different cell types, including *stromal* tissue, which consists of smooth muscle and connective tissue cells, and *glandular* tissue, which consists of epithelial cells. Epithelial cells line and secrete fluid into a network of prostatic ducts. Epithelial cells also give rise to prostate cancer.

Terminating in the prostatic urethra, a series of twenty ducts subdivide and permeate the prostate gland. At the end of each duct are balloon-like outpouchings called *acini.* These ducts drain the prostate and dump their secretions into the urethra. If these acini or ducts become blocked, they become distended, causing pain and inflammation.

The ducts that drain the central zone enter the prostatic urethra at an oblique angle, opposite the flow of urine from the bladder. This configuration creates a valve-like arrangement that prevents urine from refluxing into the ducts during urination. (During urination, if there is a restriction to flow, urine can backwash into the prostatic ducts.)

Ducts that drain the peripheral zone pursue a tortuous route before entering the urethra. As a result, they are more likely to cause plumbing problems resulting from clogs in the line. When they finally enter the urethra, they do so at a horizontal angle or, in some cases, at an angle aligned directly into the flow of urine. Consequently, urine can easily reflux into these ducts. This explains why prostatitis usually arises within the peripheral zone of the prostate. I'll expand this concept when we discuss prostatitis in Chapter 3.

EARLY PROSTATE DEVELOPMENT

At the time of birth, the prostate measures the size of a pea. The prostate then takes a snooze until the onset of puberty. During puberty, an alarm goes off in response to an influx of testosterone (male hormone), and the prostate starts to grow.

Testosterone is manufactured by the testicles and to a lesser degree by the adrenal glands—small wafer-sized organs that rest on top of the kidneys. These organs release testosterone into the bloodstream. Classified as a messenger molecule, testosterone carries a coded message that stimulates prostate cell growth. In order to deliver its message, testosterone first attaches itself to a special receptor that is located on the outside surface of the prostate cell. This docking maneuver unlocks a door that allows testosterone to float inside the prostate cell. Once inside, a special enzyme, called *5-alpha reductase*, latches onto the testosterone molecule and decodes the message by converting testosterone into *dihydrotestosterone*, a hormone-like substance that is ten times more potent than testosterone.

Dihydrotestosterone stimulates prostate cell growth by activating special molecules called growth factors. Growth factors program prostate cells to start making copies of themselves. Other molecules, called antigrowth factors, try to prevent a population explosion by coaxing older prostate cells to commit suicide (a process called *apoptosis*). From the onset of puberty until a man reaches the age of thirty, growth factors outperform antigrowth factors and the prostate gets bigger, eventually reaching the size of a golf ball. After the age of thirty, equilibrium is established between cell growth and cell death, and the prostate takes another snooze and stops growing, at least for a while. For some men, it receives another wake-up call, which can lead to problems such as *benign prostatic hypertrophy* (BPH), which will be discussed in Chapter 2.

Prostate Function

Now that we've covered the basics of prostate anatomy, let's explore how the prostate affects urinary and reproductive function. Since it's situated at the intersection of the urinary and reproductive superhighways, a prostate breakdown can create a traffic jam in both directions.

URINARY TRACT

We'll start with the urinary tract first. As the bladder fills with urine, it stretches. In an adult, the bladder can comfortably hold twelve ounces of urine without discomfort. As the bladder fills, nerves that travel from the bladder to the brain and spinal cord relay messages about the degree of bladder fullness. In response, nerves traveling in the other direction instruct the prostate and bladder neck to contract, thereby preventing urine from leaking into the prostatic urethra. Under normal circumstances, the bladder is well behaved and doesn't start contracting until it's given a go-ahead signal. At the appropriate time, urination begins when the bladder contracts and muscles in the bladder neck, prostate, and external striated sphincter relax. However, urine doesn't start flowing until the bladder pressure exceeds the urethral pressure, and it stops whenever the situation is reversed. At the end of urination, urethral muscular contractions milk the last few drops of urine trapped inside the prostatic urethra back into the bladder.

When the prostatic urethra is obstructed, though, it's a different story: The passage of urine becomes difficult, or even impossible. In addition, urethral obstruction can cause urinary reflux into the prostate, setting the stage for prostatitis.

SEXUAL FUNCTION

The prostate also has an important role in sexual function. Secretions made by prostate epithelial cells supply hungry sperm with nutrients; protect sperm by neutralizing acidic vaginal secretions; liquefy seminal fluid once it's reached its destination; and cause the cervix to relax, clearing the way for sperm to begin their marathon swim.

The prostate is also intimately involved in the events surrounding ejaculation. Just prior to orgasm, things happen in a hurry. To begin with, when the testicles receive the message that things are about to explode, they team up with their buddies, the paired *epididymides* and *vasa* (see Figure 1), and start contracting. Their contractions push "sperm-in-waiting" into a holding area at the opening of the ejaculatory duct, just outside the prostate. Simultaneously, the paired seminal vesicles begin contracting and bathe the newly arrived sperm with a tasty meal of sugary fluid (about a teaspoon). The sperm have to eat their meal on the run, though, since they're immediately propelled through the ejaculatory duct into the prostatic urethra. Meanwhile, the bladder neck slams shut, thus preventing the loss of seminal fluid into the bladder. At the same time, the prostate contracts and empties its contents, about a tablespoon of fluid, into the prostatic urethra. As these three fluids are mixed together, the prostatic urethra creates an ejection chamber by contracting against a closed external striated sphincter. When mission control receives the signal that all systems are "go" and the countdown begins, the pelvic floor muscles start rhythmic contractions. At the point of no return, the external striated sphincter suddenly relaxes, and you have, well, "liftoff."

As we'll learn in the chapters that follow, if the prostate is diseased, it can have a negative effect on fertility and sexual function. For instance, prostatic inflammation or infection can cause infertility, painful ejaculation, or even impotence (failure to achieve an erection). Furthermore, prostate cancer can also cause impotence by disrupting the nerves that cause an erection, or it can cause blood in the ejaculate by invading the seminal vesicles.

The prostatic secretions also play an important role in preventing prostate infection. Made continuously, prostatic secretions flush foreign debris and bacteria from inside the prostate into the prostatic urethra and secrete a substance called *antibacterial factor* that kills bacteria on contact (see page 61).

Finally, in case you're wondering, men can function normally without a prostate. That is, they still can have normal urination and sexual function (but not fertility, since there isn't any fluid released during ejaculation). Furthermore, after a vasectomy, men can still ejaculate seminal fluid; it just won't contain any sperm.

Conclusion

Although much maligned, your prostate doesn't have to make you *prostrate* (laid low). Now that you have a basic understanding of prostate anatomy and physiology, I'll teach you how to maintain optimal prostate health.

2

Prostate Enlargement: Benign Prostatic Hyperplasia (BPH)

Prostate enlargement is the result of a condition known as *benign prostatic hyperplasia,* commonly referred to as BPH. It is the most common benign tumor in men over the age of sixty. The term *benign* means that there aren't any cancer cells present; *prostatic* refers to the prostate; and *hyperplasia* means that the prostate is enlarged due to an increased number of prostate cells.

BPH has plagued men throughout recorded history. Until the advent of modern medicine, BPH was primarily treated with natural therapies. It wasn't until the nineteenth century, when anesthesia became available, that doctors began to substitute surgical therapies for natural ones. Another century passed before effective BPH medical therapies were discovered in the 1970s. Since then, a growing list of BPH therapies has become available.

In the first part of this chapter, I'll share new insights that have emerged over the past quarter-century regarding the incidence, causes, symptoms, and state-of-the-art treatments for BPH. Then I'll suggest natural therapies that have proven effective in treating symptomatic BPH.

Types of BPH

BPH can be subdivided into three categories: microscopic, macroscopic, and clinical. The number of men that have BPH within each of these categories varies according to age.

MICROSCOPIC BPH

Microscopic BPH refers to changes that can be seen only under the microscope. When viewed this way, BPH appears like swirls of tissue that are made of three different cell types. These cell types include glandular cells that secrete fluid; smooth muscle cells that make the prostate contract; and connective tissue that holds the other two cell types together. Although BPH is considered by many to be an "old man's disease," researchers have discovered that 20 percent of men in their forties have microscopic BPH. Thereafter, the incidence continues to rise. In fact, by the time men reach the age of eighty, approximately 90 percent of them will have microscopic BPH; if they live long enough, the figure approaches 100 percent. As disturbing as this sounds, two-thirds of these men won't require any treatment for their BPH. Even so, more men over the age of sixty-five are operated on each year for BPH than for any other medical condition except cataracts.

MACROSCOPIC BPH

The second category, *macroscopic* BPH ("macro" means large), refers to prostate enlargement that can either be seen with the naked eye or felt by performing a digital rectal exam. When an enlarged prostate gland is surgically removed and sliced open, BPH looks like kernels of corn (called nodules) that are clustered together in the midportion of the prostate. As BPH nodules enlarge, they have a nasty habit of pushing their neighbors out of the way. As a result, normal-appearing prostate tissue gets pushed to the outside border of the prostate. There is a limit, though, to how far prostate tissue can be pushed around, since a tough fibrous lining surrounding the prostate, called the *prostate capsule,* prevents further expansion outward. Prostate tissue that gets pushed against the prostate capsule can be felt by performing a digital rectal exam. The prostate gland lies just outside the anterior wall (abdominal side) of the rectum. Although it's only a crude estimate of the true prostate size, doctors formulate their impression of the overall prostate size based on the findings of a digital rectal examination. In the final analysis, about half of the men with microscopic BPH will develop prostate enlargement (macroscopic BPH).

CLINICAL BPH

The third category, *clinical* BPH, refers to BPH that causes urinary symptoms. Both microscopic and macroscopic BPH can cause such urinary symptoms if they block the flow of urine. Urinary symptoms come in two varieties—those that relate to voiding problems (such as a weak urinary stream) and those that relate to storage (or bladder) problems (such as a sudden, uncontrollable urge to urinate). The incidence of clinical BPH increases with age. By age fifty-five, approximately 25 percent of men complain of BPH symptoms. By age seventy-five, the figure increases to 50 percent.

Evolution of BPH

BPH has received a bum wrap over the years—it's blamed any time there's a problem with the waterworks. More often than not, this blame is undeserved. For instance, men usually assume that an enlarged prostate accounts for their frequent, nightly trips to the bathroom. Although their prostate glands may deserve part of the blame, other conditions are just as likely to be the problem (see "Causes of Nocturia" on page 27). Men also assume that if they have an enlarged prostate, it will cause urinary symptoms. Although they may be right—men with enlarged prostates have three times as many urinary symptoms as men with normal-sized prostates—size alone is not the final determiner. In fact, it is not unusual for men with significantly enlarged prostates to be completely free of urinary symptoms.

In Chapter 1 we covered prostate growth in its early years. We learned that the prostate needs male hormone to develop. Male hormone, which is converted to dihydrotestosterone inside the prostate cell, works by activating a series of growth factors that cause prostate growth. Antigrowth factors counterbalance prostate growth by coaxing aging prostate cells to die early. Now let's take a closer look at prostate growth during its formidable years.

Starting around age forty, the prostate starts growing again. Although the exact mechanism that triggers this wake-up call is unknown, recent insights have begun to emerge. Based on scientific research, scientists have concluded that a combination of factors—including genetic, environmental, dietary, and hormonal influences—conspire to reawaken dormant prostate cells. Of all these factors, testosterone appears to be the most important: Men that lack this male hormone don't develop BPH. Estrogen, a close cousin of testosterone, also plays a role. Although it is a female hormone, the testicles and other tissues in the body make small amounts of estrogen. Like testosterone, estrogen is a messenger molecule that stimulates prostate growth factors.

What we do know about this renewed growth cycle is that it is confined to a small area called the *transitional zone* (see Chapter 1). In a normal-sized prostate, the transitional zone accounts for only 5 percent of the total prostate volume. However, in BPH the transitional zone expands significantly, sometimes becoming as large as a grapefruit (see Figure 2.1 on page 23). Just the same, as long as the newly formed tissue has room to grow, it behaves itself and doesn't obstruct the flow of urine. Yet, if it runs out of space, the displaced tissue becomes unruly and starts pushing back. When this happens it starts to squeeze the urethra shut and clogs up the waterworks. The urethra—which is normally the size of a crayon—becomes compressed to the size of a cocktail straw or smaller.

Size isn't the only thing that matters. When the hyperplastic tissue starts flexing its muscles, the increase in muscle tone can also restrict the flow of urine.

The prostate's composition also accounts for some of its behavior. Normally, the prostate is composed of 40 percent smooth muscle tissue, 20 percent glandular tissue, and 40 percent connective tissue. As the prostate enlarges, though, one tissue type predominates. For example, in younger

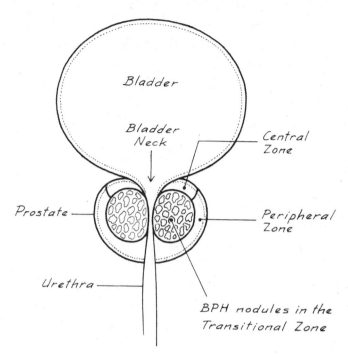

FIGURE 2.1 *Zonal Anatomy Showing BPH*

men, the ratio of stromal to epithelial tissue is 2:1, whereas in BPH it's often 5:1. It's important to determine which type predominates, since each tissue type causes prostatic obstruction in a different manner. For instance, stromal tissue is composed of smooth muscle and supportive connective tissue. Smooth muscle increases pressure within the prostate by contracting, while the elastic nature of stromal connective tissue, like a taut rubber band, accounts for its increased pressure. Although obstruction is the end result in both cases, the treatment is different (see below). Finally, excess glandular tissue creates an obstruction by sheer virtue of its size.

Individual medical therapies relieve BPH-related obstruction by either shrinking excessive glandular tissue or relaxing smooth muscle contraction, but not both. We'll explore these methods later in this chapter.

BPH Symptoms

Although the mechanism is different, excessive glandular tissue or increased smooth muscle tone can obstruct the smooth flow of urine. When this happens, men experience a variety of bothersome urinary symptoms that are called *obstructive* voiding symptoms. Other annoying urinary symptoms, called *irritative* voiding symptoms, originate in the bladder as a consequence of urethral obstruction.

OBSTRUCTIVE VOIDING SYMPTOMS

During normal urination, the prostatic urethra and external urethral sphincter (the muscle used to start and stop urination) relax, and the bladder forcefully expels urine until it's empty. Things change, though, when the prostatic urethra becomes obstructed. At first, the bladder compensates for the obstruction by working harder. Although this works for a while, problems start to develop if the obstruction persists. Backward pressure created by prostatic obstruction causes a variety of obstructive voiding complaints, which are listed below.

Dribbling of Urine

The bladder normally continues contracting until all the urine is expelled. If the prostatic urethra is obstructed, though, the bladder needs to take a breather before it can complete the job. After a short rest, the bladder starts contracting again. Consequently, urine can continue dribbling out for a minute or longer after the main flow of urine has stopped.

Terminal dribbling of urine may be unrelated to prostatic obstruction. For instance, annoying wet spots on men's trousers that appear after they've finished urinating are usually not due to BPH. Instead, drops of urine that become trapped within the urethra (where it's compressed against the trouser's "fly") cause these spots. Urine dribbles out once this pressure is relieved. Men can avert this problem by simply pulling down their pants to urinate instead of using their flies.

Split Urinary Stream

A split urinary stream is another frequent complaint that is unrelated to BPH. Instead, a split urinary stream occurs when the two edges of the urethral meatus (where the urine comes out the tip of the penis) become stuck together. Urine is diverted in two directions until the force of the urinary stream forces the two edges apart. In the meantime, urine goes everywhere. To correct this problem, simply place a thumb tip on each side of the urethral meatus and gently spread the lips apart before urinating.

Weak Stream

Men with BPH frequently complain of a weak urinary stream. They often joke that they're no longer able to write their names in the snow (or sand). Narrowing of the prostatic urethra usually accounts for this complaint. However, a tuckered-out bladder can also cause a weak urinary stream.

Intermittent Urination

Men with obstructive BPH often complain that they have to start and stop a number of times before they can empty their bladder. This happens because the bladder needs to take a breather several times during urination.

Hesitant Urination

If the prostatic urethra is obstructed, the bladder needs to get a running start before it can overcome the blockage. This pressure buildup can take thirty seconds or longer. Men also complain that they have to strain or bear down in order to urinate.

A "bashful" bladder can also cause hesitant urination. Although the result is the same—delay at the starting gate—a bashful bladder is caused by self-consciousness when "under the gun" at the urinal, not obstruction. Voiding in the privacy of an enclosed stall will normally rectify this situation.

Sensation of Incomplete Emptying

Men with BPH often complain that no sooner have they zipped up their trousers and walked away from the toilet than they have the urge to urinate again. They're often surprised at the amount of urine that comes out the second time around. This happens because the bladder doesn't empty itself during the first go-round. Men may also experience a dull fullness sensation in their lower abdomen just above the pubic bone, where the bladder is located. This fullness sensation is caused by retained urine.

If men are unable to empty their bladder completely, they develop *urinary retention*. Urinary retention can be either acute or chronic. As the name implies, *acute* urinary retention comes on quickly. Any man who has ever experienced this condition will tell you that it's an emergency. An acutely distended bladder is extremely painful.

Chronic urinary retention, on the other hand, develops more slowly and is usually not painful. In fact, men are often unaware that they are in retention until they develop *overflow incontinence*. Just as the name implies, overflow incontinence occurs when urine overflows an already too-full bladder. Bed-wetting in older men is usually due to overflow incontinence.

IRRITATIVE VOIDING SYMPTOMS

Irritiative voiding symptoms are bladder-related urinary symptoms that develop secondary to prostatic obstruction. Under normal circumstances, the pressure within the bladder remains low as it fills with urine. Once the bladder is full, it relays a signal to the brain that prompts a response. We can respond by stopping what we are doing and heading to the bathroom, or we can choose to delay urination. If we choose to urinate, the first step is to relax the external urethral sphincter and prostatic urethra. This maneuver signals the bladder to start contracting. Once the bladder pressure exceeds the urethral pressure, urine enters the urethra and flows to the outside.

If the prostatic urethra is obstructed, however, the bladder has to work harder to overcome increased urethral pressure. It does this by developing more muscle tissue. Just as weight lifting develops stronger muscles, a "bladder workout" does the same thing. Unfortunately, the end result is not the same. Unlike stronger biceps muscles (which become more efficient as they thicken), bladder muscle becomes less efficient as it thickens. That's because bladder muscle becomes infiltrated with scar tissue as it thickens. In contrast to normal bladder tissue, scar tissue doesn't stretch. As a result, a thickened bladder becomes smaller and less elastic. A thickened bladder also loses the ability to accommodate urine without increasing the pressure as it fills. Therefore, a thickened bladder creates increased backward pressure on the kidneys. Ultimately, if this backward pressure becomes high enough, it can cause renal failure (kidney shutdown). Men with thickened bladders often complain of the following voiding symptoms:

Frequent Urination

A small, thickened bladder holds less urine. Therefore, men with thickened bladders void more frequently (especially if their bladders don't empty completely).

Urgent Urination

A thickened, muscular bladder operates on a hair trigger: The least little thing—running water, for instance—can cause it to fire without warning.

Nocturia

Nocturia means getting up at least twice during the night to urinate. The combination of incomplete bladder emptying coupled with a smaller-than-normal bladder capacity means frequent trips to the bathroom throughout the night. Nocturia can also be caused by problems other than BPH. (See "Causes of Nocturia" on page 28.)

Urinary Incontinence

A thickened bladder can cause an involuntary loss of urine. Forceful bladder contractions can overpower urethral resistance within a matter of seconds. As a result, men often wet their pants before they can make it to the bathroom.

PROGRESSION OF SYMPTOMS

Scientific research has revealed that BPH-related symptoms can improve, remain stable, or worsen with time. In one study, for four years researchers followed 500 men with varying degrees of prostate symptoms. Based on the results of a voiding questionnaire called the International Prostate Symp-

Causes of Nocturia

Nocturia, or frequent nighttime urination, affects the majority (72 percent) of elderly adults, one quarter of whom get up to urinate three or more times nightly. Most men assume (incorrectly) that their prostate is to blame. Although BPH can cause nocturia, it is usually a result of one or more of the following conditions:

- medications (particularly diuretics—"water pills")
- medical conditions (i.e., diabetes mellitus, stroke, renal disease, and heart disease)
- sleep apnea
- periodic leg movements
- excessive fluid intake before bedtime
- alcoholic and caffeinated beverages
- leg swelling due to excess fluid collection
- excess salt loss in the urine
- excessive nocturnal urinary output (due to a lack of vasopressin—a hormone produced by the brain that normally slows down nighttime urinary output)

A thorough medical evaluation will often pinpoint the cause of nocturia. You can help your doctor by keeping a *voiding diary* (see page 30). You can also reduce your nightly forays to the bathroom by:

- limiting fluid intake after dinnertime
- changing or timing of medication (for instance, taking fluid pills in the afternoon rather than at nighttime)
- wearing support stocking and taking afternoon naps (this helps mobilize fluid from the lower legs during the day rather than during the night)
- eliminating alcoholic and caffeinated beverages[1]

tom Score (commonly referred to as I-PSS; see page 31), these men were divided into three groups—those with mild, moderate, and severe symptoms. Although the goal of these studies was not to see how long treatment could be delayed, after four years or more, the majority of men with mild to moderate voiding symptoms either improved or remained stable.[2]

Five other scientific studies have shown that the majority of men with moderate symptoms (I-PSS from eight to nineteen) who were followed for five years either improved (40 percent) or remained stable (45 percent); only 15 percent became worse.[3]

A number of men with *severe* voiding symptoms who were left alone however, got into trouble. We'll now explore how urologists differentiate between these two groups.

Diagnosis of BPH

Even though BPH is the most common condition affecting the prostate, the majority of men with BPH are either asymptomatic or have mild symptoms. As discussed above, the majority of these men don't require any further treatment.

On the other hand, some men with moderate BPH symptoms, and most men with severe BPH symptoms, if left untreated, are at risk of developing BPH-related medical problems (such as progressive bladder or kidney damage).

Differentiating between BPH that deserves further evaluation and treatment and BPH that doesn't requires a thorough medical evaluation. Your doctor's evaluation should include:

- taking a detailed history
- analyzing a symptom score questionnaire
- performing a physical examination
- evaluating a urinalysis
- ordering a blood study

TAKING A DETAILED HISTORY
Men with urinary difficulties often assume that their problem is due to an enlarged prostate. Other men assume that their urinary symptoms

are a natural consequence of getting older. Both of these assumptions are often wrong. Other conditions frequently cause BPH-type urinary symptoms.

Therefore, if you are experiencing voiding difficulties, make an appointment with your physician. So you won't forget anything, make a list of your voiding complaints. When you come in for your appointment, bring a copy for your physician.

I also suggest keeping a *voiding diary*—that is, a log that itemizes your voiding history. Record the frequency and amount of urination plus the amount and timing of your fluid intake throughout the day. Be sure to jot down any specific urinary complaints next to the time that they occur. Record your voiding habits for a week. This diary will give your doctor a more accurate picture of your urinary difficulties.

INTERNATIONAL PROSTATE SYMPTOM SCORE (I-PSS) QUESTIONNAIRE

In addition to going over your list of questions and analyzing your voiding diary, your doctor should ask you some additional questions about your voiding habits. You should be asked to fill out an International Prostate Symptom Score (I-PSS) questionnaire (see page 31). Your symptom score will be used to determine whether you have mild, moderate, or severe BPH symptoms. This score will help your physician determine if you need additional evaluation and treatment.

BPH can cause a variety of lower urinary tract symptoms. The term *lower urinary tract* refers to the bladder, prostate, and urethra. As mentioned above, irritative voiding symptoms are usually bladder-related, whereas obstructive voiding symptoms are usually prostate-related.

The International Prostate Symptom Score consists of a series of questions about seven lower urinary tract symptoms. The severity of each of these symptoms is measured on a scale of 0 to 5, as listed below. The scores of the seven categories are then added together to give a symptom score. The maximum score is 35. Men with scores of 0 to 7 have *mild* voiding symptoms; those with scores of 8 to 19 have *moderate* voiding symptoms; and those with scores above 20 have *severe* voiding symptoms.

INTERNATIONAL PROSTATE SYMPTOM SCORE (I-PSS)

	Not at all	Less than 1 time in 5	Less than 1/2 the time	About 1/2 the time	More than 1/2 the time	Almost always	Your Score
1. Incomplete Emptying Over the past month, how often have you had a sensation of not emptying your bladder completely after you finished urinating?	0	1	2	3	4	5	
2. Frequency Over the past month, how often have you had to urinate again less than two hours after you finished urinating?	0	1	2	3	4	5	
3. Intermittency Over the past month, how often have you found you stopped and started again several times when you urinated?	0	1	2	3	4	5	
4. Urgency Over the past month, how often have you found it difficult to postpone urination?	0	1	2	3	4	5	
5. Weak Stream Over the past month, how often have you had a weak urinary stream?	0	1	2	3	4	5	
6. Straining Over the past month, how often have you had to strain or push to begin urination?	0	1	2	3	4	5	
	Not at all	1 time	2 times	3 times	4 times	+5 times	
7. Nocturia Over the past month, how many times did you most typically get up to urinate from the time you went to bed at night until the time you got up in the morning?	0	1	2	3	4	5	

TOTAL I-PSS SCORE _____

QUALITY OF LIFE DUE TO URINARY SYMPTOMS

	Not at all	Pleased	Mostly satisfied	Mixed	Mostly dissatisfied	Unhappy	Terrible
If you were to spend the rest of your life with your urinary condition just the way it is now, how would you feel about it?	0	1	2	3	4	5	6

Reprinted with permission.
K. Ezz El Din, "The Correlation Between Bladder Outlet Obstruction and Lower Urinary Tract Symptoms As Measured by the International Prostate Symptom Score," *Journal of Urology* 156 (September 1996): 1024.

These scores are used to assess symptom severity. However, they should not be used to diagnose BPH alone, as other conditions can cause similar complaints.

CONDITIONS THAT MIMIC BPH

A variety of conditions can cause voiding symptoms that are similar to BPH. A careful history, thorough physical examination, and selective tests can usually differentiate between these conditions and BPH. Conditions that can mimic BPH include:

- urethral stricture (scar tissue)
- a bladder stone or stone in the distal ureter (just before it enters the bladder)
- bladder, prostate, or urethral cancer
- bladder, prostate, or urethral infection
- neurological diseases such as Parkinson's disease, multiple sclerosis, or stroke
- medical diseases such as diabetes
- excessive fluid intake
- normal voiding changes associated with aging

PERFORMING A PHYSICAL EXAMINATION

A physical examination allows a physician to detect BPH-related findings—for example, an enlarged prostate or a distended bladder. Therefore, every BPH evaluation should include a digital rectal examination (see Figure 2.2 on page 33) and an evaluation of the lower abdomen where the bladder is located.

The prostate is located anteriorly (on the abdominal side), just above the rectum, approximately three inches inside the rectum from the anus. Normally, the prostate measures about the size of a walnut (approximately 25 cubic centimeters). However, an enlarged prostate may measure as big as a tennis ball (50 cubic centimeters) or bigger. The surface of the prostate should be smooth and uniform and have a consistency similar

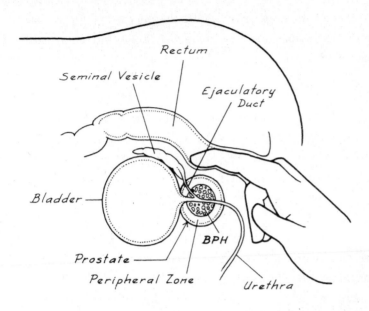

FIGURE 2.2 *Digital Rectal Examination*

to that of the tip of the nose. If the prostate feels abnormal, further investigation is warranted.

A distended bladder can be felt by thumping the lower abdomen, just above the pubic bone. This technique is similar to the one that savvy grocery shoppers use to determine whether a melon is ripe or not. They tap the skin of the melon with their finger and listen to the sound it makes. Similarly, the bladder is tapped with the middle finger of one hand (the dominant hand) against the middle finger of the other hand. The stationary finger is positioned flat against the abdominal skin overlying the bladder. If the bladder is empty, it emits a hollow sound; if the bladder is full, a dull sound is heard. If the bladder is still distended after voiding, or if you are unable to urinate, further evaluation and treatment will be necessary.

EVALUATING A URINALYSIS

The term *urinalysis* literally means analysis of the urine. A dipstick is used to check a urine sample for any signs of protein, sugar, blood, or infection.

The urine is then examined under the microscope for any other abnormalities. If an abnormality is found on either examination, further testing may be indicated.

ORDERING A BLOOD STUDY

A *prostate specific antigen* (PSA) blood test is routinely ordered to evaluate BPH-related symptoms. PSA screens for prostate cancer (see page 115). If the PSA result is abnormal, further testing may be necessary.

ADDITIONAL TESTS

If the International Prostate Symptom Score is less than 8, the five steps listed above are all that are necessary. However, if the score is 8 or above (indicating that the symptoms are moderate or severe), your physician may suggest some of the following additional tests before making any treatment recommendations:

Renal and Bladder Ultrasound

Your doctor may order a renal and bladder ultrasound. Performed on outpatients, this simple noninvasive test uses harmless sound waves to detect any kidney or bladder abnormalities.

Urodynamic Test

Your doctor may also perform a urodynamic test. This test helps differentiate between bladder and prostate-related voiding problems. Performed on an outpatient basis in the hospital or a doctor's office, a urodynamic study measures bladder and prostatic urethral pressures as the bladder fills with fluid, and again during urination. This is done with a tiny catheter equipped with tiny transducers that is gently inserted into the urethra all the way through to the bladder, and with several electrodes placed on either side of the anus. Information obtained from a urodynamic test can help predict the cause and severity of urinary obstruction.

Conventional Treatments for BPH

When considering BPH treatment options, factors that need to be considered include the size of the prostate gland, the coexistence of other medical problems, and your expectations of a successful treatment outcome. In addition, other treatment-related issues such as side effects, cost, success rate, and time out of work need to be addressed.

Traditionally, in conventional medicine, men with symptomatic BPH are treated with watchful waiting, medical therapy, surgical therapy, or a combination of the three.

WATCHFUL WAITING

Watchful waiting, as the name implies, means that men are watching rather than treating their BPH symptoms. Watchful waiting has a number of advantages and disadvantages. Advantages include:

Lower Cost

Other than a yearly doctor visit and a few blood tests, nothing else is required. Watchful waiting also avoids the cost of BPH-related medications and surgery, which can be very expensive. This cost multiplies, since BPH medications must be taken indefinitely—if they're stopped prematurely, annoying urinary symptoms tend to reoccur. Surgery is obviously even more expensive (at least initially).

No Side Effects

BPH medications and surgery can cause a number of unpleasant side effects. For instance, medications can cause fatigue, dizziness, and impotence. Surgery has its share of side effects as well. These can include impotence, urinary incontinence, and bleeding.

No Unnecessary Treatment

Finally, watchful waiting avoids treating men that don't need to be treated. This usually pertains to men with mild to moderate voiding symptoms. Most of these voiding symptoms will either remain stable or improve over time.

Contraindications to Watchful Waiting

Watchful waiting is not recommended for men with severe urinary symptoms (I-PSS greater than 20). The risk of permanent damage to the kidneys or bladder is greatest for men with severe urinary symptoms. Watchful waiting, instead of definitive medical or surgical treatments, may allow the bladder to permanently lose its tone (ability to empty), thereby rendering subsequent treatments ineffective. In addition, watchful waiting may allow underlying conditions to go undiagnosed and untreated. Therefore, watchful waiting is not recommended, regardless of the symptoms, if you have any of the *contraindications,* or conditions, listed below.

Urinary Retention If the bladder becomes distended, it can lose the ability to contract. Therefore, if urinary retention isn't treated immediately, the bladder can suffer permanent damage. As a result, a permanent catheter may be needed to drain the bladder.

Incomplete Bladder Emptying If the bladder is distended on physical examination, or if you are unable to sufficiently empty your bladder (the amount left in the bladder is ten ounces or more), definitive treatment, rather than watchful waiting, is the appropriate therapy.

Renal Insufficiency Prostatic obstruction can cause significant backward pressure in the bladder. This pressure is transmitted from the bladder to the kidneys. As a result, kidney function may become impaired. Failure to relieve the obstruction in time can result in permanent kidney damage.

Recurrent Hematuria Hematuria means blood in the urine. While many other conditions can cause hematuria, BPH is the most common cause of hematuria in males.

Recurrent Urinary Tract Infections Due to BPH Urinary tract infections are unusual in men under the age of forty. However, after the age of forty, the reverse is true; the incidence of male urinary tract infection increases. BPH-related urinary obstruction contributes to this age-related difference in infection rates.

Bladder Stones Urine routinely contains crystals that are flushed to the outside during urination. However, if the bladder doesn't empty completely, crystals often settle to the bottom of the bladder, stick together, and form bladder stones. Unlike kidney stones, bladder stones rarely pass—they have trouble making it over the hump of an enlarged prostate. Consequently, as crystals continue to accumulate, bladder stones continue to enlarge. If left unattended, a bladder stone can become as large as a softball.

Bladder Diverticulum Urinary obstruction compels the bladder to push harder to overcome the blockage. If the pressure becomes great enough, it can cause part of the inner lining of the bladder to herniate (poke through) the wall of the bladder to the outside. This pocket of bladder tissue (called a bladder diverticulum) acts like a pop-off valve for the bladder: Every time the bladder contracts, the diverticulum balloons out. If the obstruction becomes worse, the diverticulum offsets the increase in bladder pressure by enlarging. Ultimately, a diverticulum can become as large as the bladder. This creates other problems. Unlike the bladder, a bladder diverticulum lacks any muscular tissue—it's made up of flimsy bladder lining (therefore, it can't contract). Consequently, urine becomes trapped, thereby increasing the risk of recurrent urinary tract infections and bladder stones.

MINIMIZING URINARY SYMPTOMS

Although watchful waiting means that drugs and surgery aren't on the agenda, it doesn't mean that you shouldn't take whatever steps are necessary to help reduce or minimize BPH symptoms. In fact, some very simple measures—which are entirely free and without side effects—can reduce or eliminate many of the annoying BPH-related urinary symptoms.

Avoid certain beverages and food items that contain caffeine. Coffee, tea, soda, and chocolate are all examples. Alcohol can also provoke involuntary bladder contractions. Reduce drinking after dinner, to help trim those nighttime trips to the bathroom.

Decongestants (e.g., brand name Sudafed®), antihistamines (e.g., Benadryl®), and over-the-counter sleep medications (e.g., NyQuil®) can cause serious problems for men with BPH because they can completely shut off the flow of urine. Other prescription medications (particularly antidepressant medication) have the same effect. Therefore, if you have any BPH-related voiding symptoms, be sure to inform your doctor and pharmacist. Also, be sure to check with them before taking any new medications.

Keep a voiding diary. If you experience an urgent need to urinate, try urinating "by the clock." It works like this: If you notice that you have a severe urge to urinate every two hours, try urinating before you get the urge. For instance, void every hour and a half (even though you don't have an urge to urinate). This way, you won't be caught by surprise. But don't delay urination if you feel the urge to urinate. When the bladder becomes overdistended, it becomes difficult (if not impossible) to urinate.

While traveling, avoid drinking excess fluids. If you're taking a car trip, plan a rest stop at least every hour or two. For emergencies, pack a sealed container under your front car seat that you can use as a makeshift urinal (plus some blindfolds and earplugs for your passengers).

As we'll discuss in the next section, natural therapies can significantly improve or eliminate bothersome urinary symptoms without the cost or side effects of medications or surgery.

MEDICAL THERAPY FOR BPH

Medical therapy, for the purposes of this discussion, involves the use of pharmaceutical drugs. The first such therapy for BPH was reported in 1969. Since then, a variety of other BPH drug therapies have become available. Medical therapies should be considered if you have moderate or severe voiding symptoms (an I-PSS of 8 to 35). You will need a thorough medical evaluation, and be prepared to follow up every six to twelve months so your physician can monitor your progress. BPH medical therapies fall into two broad categories: medications that relax prostate and bladder neck smooth muscle tissue (called *alpha-blocker therapy*) and medications that shrink the size of the prostate (called *hormonal therapy*).

Alpha-Blocker Therapy

Alpha-blockers are usually the first drugs of choice. They block smooth muscle contraction by blocking the activity of the *autonomic nervous system*. Activities that are vital to survival (such as breathing, digestive function, and cardiac function) are controlled by the autonomic nervous system. Smooth muscle contraction is caused by *alpha-adrenergic receptors,* which are responsible for processing the signals sent by the autonomic nervous system.

Researchers have discovered that prostatic smooth muscle contraction is mediated by a subgroup of alpha-receptors called *alpha-1* receptors. This discovery allowed scientists to devise medications that target these receptors more specifically, which produced fewer side effects. Currently, three FDA-approved selective alpha-1 blockers are used to treat symptomatic BPH. These are doxazosin (Cardura), terazosin (Hytrin), and tamsulosin (Flomax).

In addition to relaxing prostatic smooth muscle tissue, alpha-blockers relax smooth muscle that is located within the walls of arterial blood vessels. This dual property allows the medications doxazosin and terazosin to also treat high blood pressure. This dual function also accounts for most of the side effects that are associated with alpha-blocker medications. However, in the late 1990s, researchers formulated tamsulosin (Flomax), which targets the prostate, not the blood vessels, so that it doesn't affect blood pressure.

On the positive side, alpha-blockers improve BPH symptoms and urinary flow rate in about two-thirds of the men who take them, thereby preventing the cost and possible complications of surgery. They also can be used to treat high blood pressure. Alpha-blockers can also be taken just once a day and start working immediately, reaching their full effectiveness within a matter of weeks.

On the negative side, alpha-blocking medications are expensive, especially when you realize these drugs must be taken indefinitely. There are also some drug-induced side effects to consider. Approximately 10 percent of men experience drowsiness and headaches. A sudden drop in blood pressure with a change in position (a condition known as *postural hypotension*) occurs 5 percent of the time. Also, a small percentage of men treated with tamsulosin experience nasal congestion and delayed or retrograde ejaculation (where seminal fluid goes backward into the bladder, rather than forward into the urethra and out the penis). Fortunately, all these side effects disappear once the medication is stopped. Furthermore, the incidence of these side effects usually decreases after the medication has been taken for a while.

Hormonal Therapies

In 1984, researchers discovered that an oral medication called finasteride (brand name Proscar) blocks the conversion of testosterone to dihydrotestosterone by blocking the enzyme 5-alpha reductase. When the prostate is no longer stimulated by dihydrotestosterone, it shrinks. In fact, finasteride shrinks the size of the prostate by 20 percent or more. As you might expect, finasteride works best in men with large prostates—that is, prostates that are greater than 40 cubic centimeters (about the size of a medium tomato).

Like alpha-1 blockers, finasteride has certain benefits and drawbacks. The benefits of finasteride include an improvement in BPH symptoms in two-thirds of men who take it, and an improvement in urinary flow rate in one-third of men. In addition, scientific research has shown that long-term use of finasteride can prevent urinary retention by over 50 percent and reduce the need for prostate surgery. Finasteride also offers an unexpected bonus for men with male pattern baldness—it increases hair growth. Finally, finasteride has an excellent safety profile.

However, in spite of these benefits, finasteride does have a few drawbacks. Like alpha-blockers, finasteride must be taken indefinitely for it to work. However, unlike alpha-blockers (which act quickly), finasteride works more slowly—it must be taken for six months or more before it is known for sure whether the medication is going to be effective. It is also as expensive as alpha-blockers, and it has a few potential side effects. Approximately 5 percent of men taking finasteride experience impotence (the inability to obtain or maintain an erection), 4 percent complain of decreased sex drive, and less than 1 percent notice breast enlargement. In addition, about one-third of men experience a reduction of seminal fluid. These side effects disappear once the medication is stopped. Finally, finasteride appears to work only in men with big prostates.

There is one final point to consider: Finasteride decreases serum PSA by up to 50 percent. Therefore, before starting finasteride, men should have a baseline PSA blood test. They should then repeat another PSA blood test six months later to establish a new baseline PSA value. (Propecia, a weaker version of finasteride that is used to treat male pattern baldness, also lowers PSA readings by 50 percent.)[4]

Once a new baseline PSA value has been established, if the PSA level starts to increase (and the patient is still taking finasteride), it may be an early warning sign of prostate cancer. Whereas finasteride prevents normal prostate cells from making excess PSA, it doesn't have the same effect on prostate cancer cells.

SURGICAL THERAPIES FOR BPH

When I first started my urology training in 1978, most men with severe BPH symptoms were treated with surgery. Even though fewer surgeries are performed today, surgical therapy still offers the best long-term results for men with symptomatic BPH. Just the same, surgery is generally reserved for the following circumstances:

- when BPH symptoms aren't controlled with medical therapy
- when men forgo a trial of medical therapy and select surgery instead
- when there are contraindications to treating BPH (see page 36) with watchful waiting or medical therapies

Before considering surgical therapies for BPH, you should undergo the same evaluation as you would when considering BPH medical therapies. Then you need to consider the possibility of surgically related side effects. Although surgical therapies offer the best chance for improvement in BPH symptoms, this benefit has to be weighed against a greater risk of serious side effects, some of which are permanent. Unlike medical therapies (which are reversible), once surgery is performed, it can't be taken back.

The surgical options for treating BPH continue to expand. Some of the current therapies are less invasive than others. Although a full discussion of these therapies is beyond the scope of this book, highlights of the most popular surgical therapies are discussed below.

Transurethral Prostatectomy (TURP)

Of the men who are surgically treated for symptomatic BPH, approximately 90 percent of them will be treated with this procedure. TURP is performed through a special tube called a sheath that is inserted into the urethra. An instrument called a resectoscope is inserted into the sheath. The resectoscope holds a fiber-optic lens and a special cutting instrument called a resectoscope loop. The surgeon manipulates the loop to snip off enlarged prostate tissue. The procedure is performed under general or spinal anesthesia and takes about an hour. Men usually stay in the hospital overnight and go home the next morning. The catheter is removed in the office on the third postoperative day.

TURP is the most effective treatment for symptomatic BPH. In fact, TURP is the "gold standard" to which all other treatments are compared. It consistently improves BPH symptoms and urinary flow rates in approximately 80 percent of men, which explains why TURP accounts for the vast majority of BPH operations.

TURP can also produce complications. These include incontinence (less than 1 percent), impotence (up to 5 percent), and retrograde ejaculation (up to 90 percent). Although a TURP is initially more expensive, it is usually less expensive than a lifetime of medications.

Transurethral Incision of the Prostate

The setup for this procedure is similar to that used to perform a TURP. However, instead of whittling away prostate tissue, a special loop is used to merely cut the floor of the prostate and bladder neck. No prostate tissue is removed. The results of this procedure compare favorably with those of a TURP, and the risks are less. However, this procedure is reserved for smaller prostates—those measuring 30 cubic centimeters or less (about the size of a medium-sized plum).

Open Prostatectomy

This procedure is performed through an incision made in the lower abdomen. A knife is used to make a two-inch incision in the prostatic capsule (outer lining). The surgeon then inserts an index finger in the prostate and sweeps around the inside rim of the gland, shelling out the enlarged BPH tissue that is located just beneath the prostate capsule. To visualize this procedure, imagine cutting through the skin of a navel orange. Then stick your finger inside and sweep the orange segments loose. Finally, pluck the segments out through the hole in the orange skin.

The results and complications of this procedure compare favorably with those of a TURP. However, there is a longer hospital stay (five to seven days) and an increased risk of impotence (19 percent).

LESS INVASIVE SURGICAL PROCEDURES

The procedures described in this section are less invasive than the ones described up to this point. They are usually performed on an outpatient basis (no hospital admittance or stay) and can often be performed under local anesthesia, sometimes even in a doctor's office. However, because they are less invasive, they may also be less effective. Depending on the procedure, up to half of the men treated with minimally invasive therapies need additional surgery within five years. Many men are willing to go this route because there is a smaller chance of the previously mentioned side effects—impotence, incontinence—and no need for a blood transfusion.

Prostatic Stents

Stents are thin cage-like metal devices placed transurethrally within the prostatic urethra. Stents come in different lengths, ranging from an inch to two inches. They are initially compressed to allow them to fit through a cystoscope. The stents then spring open once they're released inside the prostatic urethra. Over a period of months, prostate tissue grows over the exposed wires and covers the stent. If this fails to occur, crystals adhere to the exposed metal surface and form stones. Exposed wires can also increase the risk of recurrent urinary tract infections.

Although stents are easy to place, they can migrate into the wrong position. Depending on the direction, they can either poke into the bladder or keep the sphincter muscle open and cause urinary incontinence. If this happens, the stents either have to be repositioned or removed.

Electrovaporization

This procedure is similar to a TURP except that a "rollerball" is used to heat prostate tissue instead of a loop that cuts the tissue. As the rollerball is pushed back and forth, electric current flows through the rollerball and vaporizes (dissolves) the prostate tissue. No tissue is removed. The chances of impotence, urinary incontinence, and retrograde ejaculation are similar to those of a TURP. The risk of bleeding, though, is less.

Laser Ablation

Lasers use high-intensity light energy of a particular wavelength to heat prostate tissue. When the temperature is high enough (at least 140° F.), tissue is *ablated* (destroyed). A variety of different laser procedures are used to treat BPH. Laser ablation of the prostate causes fewer side effects than does a TURP, but it's less effective.

Transurethral Microwave Thermotherapy

Commonly referred to as simply "microwave therapy," this procedure is performed under local anesthesia. A special urethral catheter is inserted into the urethra and emits a low-level radio-frequency energy into the prostate. Although this procedure is minimally invasive, Swedish investigators reported that more than 50 percent of men treated required additional treatment within four years. Other studies have reported that almost half of the men treated with microwave therapy developed postoperative urinary retention for up to four weeks after the procedure. Still, microwave therapy is less expensive and causes fewer side effects than does a TURP.

Transurethral Needle Ablation

A special catheter is inserted into the urethra that is equipped with needles that look like snake fangs. Once these needles pierce the prostate tissue, they emit low-level radio-frequency energy that heats the prostate. The results and side effects are similar to those of laser ablation of the prostate.

High-Intensity Focused Ultrasound

A special probe that is inserted into the rectum delivers high-intensity sound waves into the prostate. The heat generated by the ultrasound energy destroys tissue within the prostate without injuring the surrounding tissue. This procedure also has its problems. In a Japanese study, most men developed urinary retention after this procedure, and a third of the men required a TURP within three years.[5]

Natural Therapies for BPH

Plants or plant extracts have been used since ancient times to treat urinary problems. Popularly known as *phytotherapy* ("phyto" means plant), European physicians prescribe plant-derived extracts first before they resort to synthetic drugs to treat BPH. In fact, German and Austrian physicians prescribe natural therapies for mild to moderate BPH symptoms 90 percent of the time instead of synthetic medications. As further evidence of phytotherapy's popularity, Italian physicians prescribe plant extracts for symptomatic BPH nearly 50 percent of the time versus 5 percent for alpha-blockers and 5 percent for finasteride. In contrast to the United States, when European physicians write a prescription for an approved natural product, it's covered by health insurance. There are a number of reasons why European physicians use phytotherapy as a first-line treatment for BPH.

First, it costs less. A month's supply of a typical herbal extract usually costs less than a month's supply of a BPH prescription medication.

Second, phytotherapy has fewer side effects than prescription medications. Serious herbal-related side effects are extremely rare; fatal side effects are almost unheard of. The same cannot be said for prescription drugs.

Finally, phytotherapy is effective. Scientific research has shown that phytotherapy improves BPH symptoms (over placebos) in up to 70 percent of patients. Perhaps that explains why 50 percent of German urologists prefer plant-based therapies to synthetic medications for men with symptomatic BPH.

Why, then, are American urologists so reluctant to join the cause? Some doctors argue that there isn't sufficient scientific proof that herbal therapies work. Some believe that the European data are inadequate because the studies are too short in duration, the sample sizes are too small, or the studies are rarely double-blinded (where neither the patient nor the researcher knows the type of treatment being used) or placebo-controlled. American urologists attribute apparent benefits of herbal-based therapies to a placebo effect. This is understandable, since scientific studies have shown that a sugar pill alone may improve symptoms in up to 60 percent of patients.[6]

Concern about the safety of phytotherapy is another reason why American urologists discourage the use of such products. As opposed to pharmaceutical drugs—where the mechanism of action and the side effects are usually known—the mechanism of action of many phytotherapeutic products is unproven. Therefore, it may be difficult to accurately predict adverse herb-drug interactions.

Finally, American urologists caution against using phytotherapy because the quality of over-the-counter herbal products is unknown. They dismiss manufacturers' claims as being little more than advertising hype.

While I believe that the above criticisms are valid, I'm also aware that the picture is changing. Evidence-based scientific research supports the use of phytotherapy for symptomatic BPH. Although most of these data come from European studies, this information is starting to filter into American medical journals. In addition, research has shown that herbal products are generally safe. Specifically, there haven't been any life-threatening side effects reported due to herbal therapies for BPH. Finally, it is possible to manufacture quality herbal products. In Europe, government-endorsed herbal products must provide a certificate of analysis that guarantees the contents and purity of the product (plus the test results for bacterial, heavy metal, and pesticide contamination). A growing number of herbal companies in this country are starting to subscribe to the same high standards as their European counterparts. (See Appendix B for hints on selecting quality herbal products.)

For the reasons discussed above, I, like my European colleagues, frequently recommend phytotherapy to patients with mild to moderate BPH symptoms. At the same time, I would caution you against self-medication with natural BPH therapies until you've had a proper evaluation by a licensed physician. Finally, natural therapies should not be used to treat symptomatic BPH if there are any of the signs that contraindicate watchful waiting or medical therapies (see page 36).

Although it's not possible to change certain BPH risk factors—one's age or genetic makeup, for instance—it *is* possible to alter a variety of other factors that promote BPH. For example, scientific research has shown that unhealthy dietary, lifestyle, and environmental choices increase the incidence of symptomatic BPH, while healthy ones have the opposite effect. You can lower your risk of developing symptomatic BPH by adopting each of the following measures.

DIET

A healthy diet—one that's low in fat, meat, and dairy but high in fruits, vegetables, and fiber—can prevent symptomatic BPH. You can help to protect your prostate by making healthy choices in the foods you eat and, more important, don't eat.

Reduce Fat

High-fat, high-salt foods, like most junk food, increase the risk of BPH by stimulating prostate cell growth. Both red meat and dairy products are rich in saturated (animal) fat. Diets that are high in saturated animal fat have been shown to double the risk of prostate cancer. Commercial meat and dairy products often contain harmful estrogenic hormone and pesticide by-products that promote prostate cell growth. In addition, saturated fat provokes inflammatory changes within the prostate by causing oxidative DNA damage and excess production of inflammatory arachidonic acid by-products (see "Arachadonic Acid Cascade" on page 130). Finally, saturated fat induces BPH by raising insulin levels (the hormone that our bodies use to break down sugar). Elevated insulin levels stimulate prostate cell growth by increasing the production of a potent growth factor called *insulin-like growth factor type 1* (see page 111).

Eliminate Refined Sugar

Sugar increases the risk of BPH by stimulating prostate cell growth—it increases insulin levels and the production of inflammatory arachidonic acid by-products.

Eat More Fruits and Vegetables

Men who consume diets that are rich in fruits and vegetables are less likely to develop symptomatic BPH. Fruits and vegetables lower the risk of BPH because they are rich in lignans, a special type of fiber that intestinal bacteria metabolize to phytoestrogens (proteins that compete with and block the harmful effects of excess estrogen). Fruits and vegetables also lower "free testosterone" by increasing sex-hormone–binding globulin. (Ninety-eight percent of testosterone is bound to this globulin and other proteins in the blood. Only the unbound testosterone is "free" to stimulate BPH.) Eat at least five servings of fresh fruit and vegetables daily.

Eat Soy Protein

Phytoestrogens in soy protein block BPH by competing with serum estrogen and inhibiting the enzyme 5-alpha reductase. Eat at least two servings daily. (See page 134 for more information.)

Lower Serum Cholesterol

High levels of cholesterol in the prostate make it easier for testosterone and dihydrotestosterone to bind to prostate cell receptors, thereby turning on prostate growth factors. In addition to eating a diet that is low in fat and cholesterol, other measures that can lower serum cholesterol include the following: eating soy protein and garlic; drinking decaffeinated green tea; eliminating alcohol, tobacco products, and caffeine; and exercising regularly.

Eat Plenty of Fiber

Dietary fiber (plant material that isn't digested) decreases the risk of BPH by binding with and eliminating excess fat and hormones from the body. According to one report, men that increased dietary wheat bran by 10 percent experienced a 65 percent reduction in prostate enlargement.[7] Although the National Cancer Institute recommends eating between 25 and 35 grams of fiber daily, on average, Americans eat only 10 grams a day.

LIFESTYLE MODIFICATIONS

In addition to eating a healthy diet, healthy lifestyle choices can also reduce the odds of developing symptomatic BPH. Give your prostate and the rest of your body a break by adopting the following advice.

Exercise Regularly

Based on results from the Health Professionals Follow-up Study, regular exercise significantly lowers the risk of BPH, regardless of age. Researchers discovered that men who watched the most television and videotapes per week (forty-one hours or more) had twice the risk of developing severe obstructive BPH symptoms when compared to men who watched less than five hours per week.[8] So turn off the television set, stash your video card, and start exercising.

Stop Smoking

According to a Finnish study, men who smoke have a one-and-a-half times greater risk of developing urinary symptoms than men who never smoked.[9] Furthermore, smoke also contains cadmium—a toxic trace metal that increases the risk of prostate cancer and BPH by interfering with zinc metabolism within the prostate gland.

Lose Weight

Obese men have larger prostates. Obesity also increases the risk of prostate cancer. The body uses extra fat to make excess sex hormones.

AVOID ENVIRONMENTAL TOXINS

Pesticides and herbicides (weed killers) heighten the risk of BPH by causing DNA damage and altering hormone metabolism. *Endocrine disrupters*—substances that mimic natural hormones—also increase the incidence of BPH. Common examples include polychlorinated biphenols, or PCBs (used to make plastic, ink, electrical equipment, and electronic equipment), and plasticizers (substances used to make plastic food-wrap more pliable).

PHYTOTHERAPY FOR BPH

When preventive measures fail to stop the onset of BPH-related voiding symptoms, natural remedies can help. Many phytotherapeutic compounds are currently used to treat BPH. In general, these products are derived from eight plant species. The most common active ingredient in these compounds is derived from an extract made from dried berries of the American dwarf palm *Serenoa repens* (popularly known as *saw palmetto*). Other popular preparations that have been subjected to peer-reviewed scientific research include the following: pygeum (African plum tree, *Prunus africana,* formerly known as *Pygeum africanum)*, beta-sitosterol (compounds that are related to cholesterol), rye pollen extract (Cernilton), and stinging nettle *(Urtica dioica)*. While other substances are used to treat symptomatic BPH, their use is not supported by reliable scientific research. Therefore, the following discussion will be limited to the herbal therapies listed above.

Saw Palmetto *(Serenoa repens)*

Dubbed "the old man's friend," saw palmetto is unquestionably the world's most popular treatment for symptomatic BPH. Named after Sereno Watson, a nineteenth-century Harvard botanist, saw palmetto

(Serenoa repens) is a small palm tree that grows along the coastal south-eastern United States and the West Indies. It is occasionally referred by another botanical name, *Sabal serrulata*.

Saw palmetto's medicinal properties are attributed to its berries. Clusters of green fleshy berries develop in late spring and ripen to a bluish black by late summer. Once the berries are ripe, they're harvested and dried. The dried berries are then processed to make a variety of herbal products.

Native American Indians are credited with first discovering saw palmetto's healing properties. They used saw palmetto as a tonic (health stimulant) and as a treatment for urinary difficulties. Researchers have determined that the lipid-soluble components of saw palmetto berries account for their medicinal properties. Although exactly how saw palmetto works is still unclear, researchers theorize that it:

- inhibits 5-alpha-reductase enzyme activity, which in turn inhibits prostate cell growth
- inhibits molecules that cause swelling within the prostate
- inhibits enzymes that convert arachidonic acid into other inflammatory molecules
- blocks the action of estrogen (female hormone) and androgen (male hormone), which stimulate prostate cell growth
- blocks growth factors that send messages to the cell nuclei (command center) that are relayed to RNA (genetic material that makes new proteins needed for cell growth)
- blocks alpha-adrenergic receptors

A team of researchers compiled data from eighteen randomized controlled trials involving 2,935 men.[10] The outcome compared the effectiveness of saw palmetto versus a placebo in improving urinary symptoms. The researchers also evaluated saw palmetto's effect on the peak and mean urine flow (how fast the men were able to urinate), residual urine, prostate size, nocturia, and PSA. Overall, 74 percent of the men taking saw palmetto reported an improvement in their urinary symptons versus 51 percent of the men taking a placebo.

The researchers concluded that saw palmetto improved urinary tract symptoms and urinary flow rates in men with symptomatic BPH. It reduced residual urine and reduced nocturia by 25 percent. However, it did not reduce prostate size, nor did it alter the PSA blood test. Furthermore, the researchers observed that saw palmetto compared favorably to finasteride but had fewer side effects and cost less.

In fact, although saw palmetto can occasionally cause stomach upset, the incidence is comparable to a placebo medication. In addition, there aren't any known drug interactions or contraindications to taking saw palmetto.

Saw palmetto is available in a variety of preparations. These include dried berries, tablets that are made from ground-up dried berries, liquid tinctures, and liquid or solid extracts.

The recommended daily dose is 160 milligrams of a fat-soluble extract (standardized to contain 85 to 95 percent fatty acids and sterols), taken twice daily by men weighing less than 200 pounds, and three times daily by men over 200 pounds. Although it is often recommended that you take the daily amount of saw palmetto in divided doses, it also appears to work just as well if the entire dose is taken once daily.

Finally, be sure to buy saw palmetto from a reputable company (see Appendix B). Despite what the bottle says, many products fall short.

Pygeum *(Prunus africana)*

Pygeum is an evergreen tree that is native to the higher elevations of central and southern Africa. Reaching heights of 150 feet, the deeply fissured bark of the tree is harvested and then ground into a powder that can be used to treat symptomatic BPH. Although the first recorded use of pygeum as a natural remedy dates back to the eighteenth century, it became more widely used beginning in 1969, when European phytochemical researchers formulated a standardized solid extract called Tadenan.

Chemical analysis and pharmacological studies indicate that pygeum contains three categories of active ingredients. These ingredients include phytosterols (particularly beta-sitosterol), pentacyclic triterpenes (volatile oils), and ferulic acid esters (especially *n*-docosanol).

Most of the data regarding pygeum's effectiveness are derived from animal studies. Although exactly how pygeum works is unknown, research indicates that it:

- lowers cholesterol within the prostate (elevated cholesterol levels can trigger BPH)
- decreases inflammation within the prostate
- interferes with testosterone's effect on the prostate by reducing prolactin levels, a component that increases the intake of testosterone by prostate cells
- inhibits prostatic growth factors
- inhibits 5-alpha-reductase enzyme activity
- inhibits the activity of aromatase, an enzyme that produces excess estrogen in men as they age, which can contribute to BPH

Based on the results of twelve double-blind, placebo-controlled studies, pygeum proved to be significantly more effective than a placebo. Although most of the studies were either too short or involved too few patients to make any definite conclusions, one German study of particular note observed 269 men for sixty days.[11] Half of these men received 50 milligrams of pygeum (Tadenan) twice daily; the other half received a placebo. Overall, 67 percent of the men taking pygeum experienced an improvement in their voiding BPH symptoms versus 31 percent of men in the placebo group. However, most of the men in this study had only mild BPH symptoms, so it's difficult to draw any conclusions in men with more severe BPH symptoms.

Pygeum is extremely safe. Other than a rare incidence of gastrointestinal upset, there haven't been any reported drug interactions or serious side effects. The recommended dosage varies between 100 to 200 milligrams of a standardized extract of pygeum (containing 14 percent triterpenes and .5 percent *n*-docosanol) in divided daily doses. However, because indiscriminate harvesting of pygeum has threatened its survival, I recommend using other effective natural remedies before trying pygeum.

Beta-sitosterol

Beta-sitosterol is a plant-derived steroid that accounts for many of the beneficial effects of saw palmetto, pygeum, stinging nettle, and pumpkin seeds—herbs that are commonly used to treat BPH. Beta-sitosterol is a member of a larger family of plant steroids called phytosterols, which are related to cholesterol. (Our bodies use cholesterol to manufacture a variety of hormones, including male and female hormones.)

Although beta-sitosterol is derived from a number of plants, the type most commonly used in Europe is usually derived from the roots of the South African star grass *(Hypoxis rooperi)*. Native to South Africa, *Hypoxis rooperi* is also cultivated in South America, Australia, and Asia.

German researchers developed a standardized product (brand name Harzol) that contains 10 milligrams of beta-sitosterol. Harzol has become one of the most popular BPH treatments in Germany.

Although unproven, researchers theorize that *Hypoxis rooperi* has the same mechanism of action as saw palmetto and pygeum. The majority of studies have shown that beta-sitosterol improves BPH-related voiding symptoms. Two double-blind placebo-controlled European studies, one involving 177 men and the other 200 men, concluded that men taking beta-sitosterol experienced a significant improvement in urinary symptoms (lower I-PSS), quality of life, peak and median urinary flow, and residual volume when compared to the placebo group.[12] In fact, based on medical literature, investigators found that beta-sitosterol was just as effective as prescription alpha-blocker and finasteride medications. As expected, there was no change in prostate volume.

There are no known contraindications, drug interactions, or serious side effects due to beta-sitosterol when it is taken as directed. While Harzol isn't available in this country, other beta-sitosterol–containing products are available in health food stores or by mail order (Beachwood Canyon Naturally, 888-803-5333). Select a product that contains at least 50 percent beta-sitosterol. Follow the instructions on the package.

Cernilton

Pollen from plants that grow in southern Sweden is used to make a popular BPH remedy called Cernilton. This remedy is also used to treat men with nonbacterial prostatitis and prostate cancer. Although Cernilton is primarily used in Europe, this versatile natural remedy is becoming more popular in this country. In addition to improving the symptoms of prostatitis, researchers found that Cernilton improved BPH-related urinary symptoms. Cernilton is extracted from rye-grass pollen in a patented two-step process. Based on scientific research, Cernilton appears to work by:

- reducing urethral pressure
- causing smooth muscle relaxation by functioning as an alpha-blocker
- relaxing the external sphincter, the muscle used to voluntarily start and stop urination
- decreasing prostate swelling (in rats)
- inhibiting testosterone
- inhibiting 5-alpha reductase enzyme activity
- decreasing prostatic inflammation

In one double-blind placebo-controlled trial, 57 men were followed for six months: 31 took four tablets of Cernilton daily, while the remaining 26 took a placebo medication.[13] Overall, 69 percent of the Cernilton group reported a significant improvement in BPH symptoms versus 29 percent in the placebo group. In addition, 57 percent of the Cernilton group showed an improvement in bladder emptying versus 10 percent in the placebo group. Prostate size also decreased in the Cernilton group versus the placebo group. There was not a statistically significant difference between the Cernilton and placebo group in peak urinary flow rate, urinary hesitancy, urgency, intermittency, or terminal dribbling.

Cernilton is commercially available as a tablet or capsule (see page 85). When taken as directed, there are no contraindications, drug interactions, or serious side effects. However, men with pollen allergies should check with their physician first.

Stinging Nettle *(Urtica dioica)*

Nettle root extracts are used as a first-line BPH therapy in Germany, often in combination with other herbs, such as saw palmetto and pygeum. According researchers, stinging nettle appears to work by:

- inhibiting the attachment of sex-hormone–binding globulin, blocking the effect of estrogen and free androgen

- inhibiting aromatase activity, so plasma estrogen levels fall
- reducing inflammation

Nettle root has been extensively studied in European trials since 1980. Although the quality of the studies varies, the studies have shown that nettle root extract is more effective than placebo. A well-designed double-blind placebo-controlled German trial studied 41 men with moderately severe BPH symptoms (I-PSS 18).[14] After three months, the men who had been taking nettle extract reported twice the improvement (I-PSS scores fell from 18 to 8) as men in the placebo group (I-PSS scores fell from 17 to 12). Men treated with nettle extract also experienced an improved urinary flow. The normal daily dose is three to six grams, taken as a tablet or capsule containing 600 to 1,200 milligrams of a 5:1 dry extract, or 120 milligrams twice daily of a 10:1 extract (standardized for amino acid content). When nettle root extract is taken as directed, there are no serious side effects, drug interactions, or contraindications.

Conclusion

Benign prostatic hyperplasia is one of the most common reasons that men over the age of fifty see a urologist. In fact, if men live long enough, they will all develop BPH. Just the same, men with mild to moderate BPH symptoms can usually be treated expectantly (watched without treatment); while men with severe BPH symptoms are best managed with either drug therapies or surgery.

In contrast to their American counterparts, European urologists usually prescribe phytotherapy before resorting to drugs and surgery. Scientific research has shown that selected natural BPH therapies are as effective as prescription medications. In addition, natural therapies are less expensive and cause fewer side effects than conventional therapies.

3

Prostatitis

Prostatitis affects millions of men. In fact, as recently as 1990, prostatitis accounted for more doctor visits than either prostate enlargement or prostate cancer. Although prostatitis has received less media attention than either of these other two conditions, prostatitis is still the most common reason that men under the age of fifty (and the third most common reason that men over the age of fifty) see a urologist.

Moreover, millions of men harbor prostatitis but don't know it. According to one study, 50 percent of prostate tissue biopsies and 98 percent of prostate tissue removed for prostate enlargement showed signs of prostatitis.

Although the term *prostatitis* literally means inflammation ("itis") of the prostate, inflammation isn't always present. Neither is infection, even though most patients and many of their physicians assume that prostatitis is caused by a bacterial infection. Unfortunately, the term *prostatitis* has become a wastebasket term that physicians use to explain any undiagnosed symptom or condition that might possibly emanate from the prostate. Translated, this means that many men are often told that they have prostatitis when in fact they don't.

Although treatment guidelines can steer physicians in the right direction, in clinical practice doctors use a process of elimination, based on the results of trial-and-error therapies, to diagnose prostatitis. Only bacterial prostatitis can be diagnosed with certainty, because bacteria can be easily detected by laboratory testing. The exact cause of the remaining types of prostatitis is based more on speculation than fact.

While establishing a proper diagnosis is challenging enough, finding a cure for prostatitis is even more so. Despite the best treatment available, chronic prostatitis has a nasty habit of coming back. Although discouraging for the physician, the consequences of prostatitis for the patient can be devastating. Men suffering with prostatitis are often subjected to months (even years) of unrewarding doctor visits, expensive and invasive tests (which are usually normal), and a grocery list of medications—all to no avail.

So it's little wonder that urologists dub prostatitis the black sheep of the prostate family of diseases. Surveys have shown that prostatitis, more than any other prostate disease, is one they'd rather avoid.

Fortunately, there's reason for hope: Even the most stubborn cases of prostatitis can be helped by combining conventional therapies with natural remedies. Successful treatment, though, depends on an accurate diagnosis.

In the first half of this chapter, I'll walk you through the conventional steps that urologists use to reach the right diagnosis and then treat prostatitis. Building on this information in the second half of the chapter, I'll teach you how to alleviate the symptoms of prostatitis with natural therapies.

Types of Prostatitis

In an effort to standardize the terminology that is used to describe the different types of prostatitis, the National Institutes of Health proposes dividing prostatitis into four main categories: acute bacterial prostatitis (category I); chronic bacterial prostatitis (category II); chronic abacterial (nonbacterial) prostatitis (category III), which is subdivided into inflammatory (IIIa) and noninflammatory (IIIb) prostatitis; and asymptomatic inflammatory prostatitis (category IV).

As we explore each of these categories, you'll appreciate why urologists find prostatitis to be so challenging.

ACUTE BACTERIAL PROSTATITIS (CATEGORY I)

Compared to the other types of prostatitis, *bacterial prostatitis* is rare—it accounts for only 5 percent of the cases. Microscopic organisms called bacteria cause both types of bacterial prostatitis (categories I and II). Normally found in the digestive tract, bacteria come in two varieties—friendly and unfriendly.

In our digestive tract, bacteria are usually friendly. They help us digest food, make vitamins, and neutralize toxins. Although unfriendly bacteria also reside in the digestive tract, they account for less than 5 percent of the trillions of bacteria that reside in the intestinal tract. Nevertheless, unfriendly bacteria can cause a real ruckus. Among other things, unfriendly bacteria can disrupt normal digestive function and cause abdominal pain, bloating, and diarrhea. In fact, any time that bacteria venture outside the intestinal tract they become troublemakers.

As the name implies, *acute bacterial prostatitis* is caused by a bacterial infection that develops acutely (suddenly). Since the prostate is normally sterile (free of bacteria), any bacteria within the prostate are considered unfriendly. The prostate doesn't take kindly to foreign invaders. If bacteria trespass into the prostate, all havoc breaks loose. The prostate and the body's immune system unleash an all-out attack against the trespassers. The ensuing battle leads to the signs (like a hot and swollen prostate) and symptoms (like pelvic pain and difficult urination) of acute bacterial prostatitis. Men experience an explosive onset of voiding symptoms (such as urgent, frequent, and painful urination), fever, and chills. They rapidly become very sick. In fact, if acute bacterial prostatitis isn't treated promptly, bacteria can overwhelm the body's defense mechanisms and become a life-threatening emergency.

Causes

So where do these bacteria come from? In the case of acute bacterial prostatitis, the bacteria come from infected bladder urine or infected urethral secretions. (The urethra is the tube that carries urine from the bladder through the prostate to the outside.) Bacteria don't get a free ride, though. Our natural defenses are usually able to kill wayward bacteria on the spot.

In addition to infected bodily fluids, acute bacterial prostatitis can be caused by:

- *Manipulation of the urinary tract.* Sneaky bacteria can hitchhike from outside the urethra into the bladder when either a catheter or an instrument such as a cystoscope (a device that urologists use to "look" inside the bladder) is used.
- *Unsafe sexual practices.* Unprotected sex, such as anal intercourse, is another way that bacteria can pass through the urethra into the prostate.
- *Smooth muscle spasms.* When the smooth flow of urine is interrupted, bacteria can get backwashed into the ducts (tubes) that drain the prostate. Spasm of the sphincter muscles—the muscles that control the flow of urine—is the most common reason that the smooth flow of urination gets interrupted. (There are two sphincter muscles: the *bladder neck muscle,* which is located where the bladder meets the prostate, and the *external urethral striated sphincter muscle,* which is the muscle that's used to voluntarily stop urination. See pages 10 and 11.) Although reflux of urine into the prostate is common, it usually doesn't cause an infection unless the urine is infected.

CHRONIC BACTERIAL PROSTATITIS (CATEGORY II)

Although chronic bacterial prostatitis is more common than the acute variety, its incidence is still relatively insignificant (less than 5 percent) in comparison to nonbacterial prostatitis. Just the same, chronic bacterial prostatitis plagues men of all ages. It is usually, but not always, preceded by an acute bacterial infection. The infection becomes chronic if the body's defenses are unable to eradicate the offending bacteria. Any bacteria that survive can regroup and start multiplying again.

The presentation of chronic bacterial prostatitis is different from that of the acute version. That's because a small pocket of smoldering bacteria, not an overwhelming bacterial infection, is the cause. Therefore, chronic bacterial prostatitis isn't a medical emergency or life-threatening, but it can make your life miserable. Men with chronic bacterial prostatitis often suffer recurrent urinary tract infections, chronic pelvic pain, problems with sexual function, and a variety of voiding difficulties.

How the Prostate Defends Itself

The prostate is capable of killing most of the bacteria before they can gain a foothold. It does this with a few helpers. First is a sticky substance that the prostate uses to "slime" bacteria. Secreted by cells that line the prostatic ducts, this antibacterial fluid, called antibacterial factor, kills bacteria on contact. Researchers have determined that zinc is the active component of this fluid, and, fortunately, the prostate has the highest zinc concentration of any other tissue in the body. Unfortunately, this is not the case for men with chronic bacterial prostatitis. Their prostate zinc levels are extremely low (even though their blood zinc levels are normal). Restoring their prostate zinc levels to normal improves the odds of curing chronic bacterial prostatitis.

In addition to secreting antibacterial factor, the prostate enlists the help of the immune system to ward off bacterial interlopers. Once the bacteria have been annihilated, the prostate helps in the cleanup process by secreting additional fluid into the prostatic ducts. This fluid washes cellular debris and bacteria from the ducts and dumps them into the urethra. Urination then washes the secretions to the outside.

So far so good, but sometimes the body's defense mechanisms are unable to overcome the bacterial invaders. For instance, if the prostate's ducts become clogged, this prevents the antibacterial factor, antibiotics, and immune cells from reaching the bacteria. As a result, the prostatic ducts and surrounding prostatic tissue become infected, inflamed, and scarred, which causes chronic pelvic pain, painful ejaculation, and chronic prostate infection.

Also, debris trapped within obstructed prostatic ducts can harden and form stones. Although these stones are common in men and usually don't present any problems, they can contribute to chronic infection by interrupting the smooth flow of prostate secretions and by harboring bacteria between their layers, where they remain protected until they outgrow their quarters and move out.

Finally, the constant battle of fighting infection will eventually take its toll on the prostate. It can withstand the constant bombardment of toxins released by the immune system cells for only so long. The prostate becomes inflamed as a result. The battle continues as bacteria bring out their own line of defense, namely a thick, slimy coating called a *biofilm*. The bacteria are initially vulnerable as the biofilm's gooey surface is being laid down, but once the biofilm is complete, the protective covering becomes bulletproof, and the infection becomes chronic.

CHRONIC ABACTERIAL PROSTATITIS (CATEGORY III)

The term *abacterial* literally means without bacteria. Nevertheless, bacteria may be present, just not detectable. As discussed above, bacteria often remain hidden within the nooks and crannies of the prostate; they play a game of hide-and-seek.

While the cause of abacterial prostatitis is controversial, most experts agree that there are two types, based on the presence (category IIIa) or absence (category IIIb) of inflammation. In addition, since both of these categories of chronic prostatitis cause pelvic pain, some researchers lump them together under the name of *chronic pelvic pain syndrome*.

Although investigators have long suspected that stealth bacteria can cause "abacterial" prostatitis, it wasn't until the advent of molecular biology that they've been able to prove it. Now, by using genetic sequencing, scientists have been able to identify these shadowy organisms.

Inflammatory (Category IIIa)

Various theories have been proposed over the years to explain the cause of category IIIa prostatitis. As mentioned above, it may be due to an occult bacterial infection that can't be detected. Although unproven, other theories include genetic factors, hormonal imbalance, aging, chemical irritants, fungal infections, and an autoimmune response (where the body makes antibodies against itself). In the final analysis, though, the exact origin of chronic prostatitis remains elusive in most cases.

Inflammation is detected by the presence of leukocytes (a special type of white blood cell) within the prostatic secretions. (See How Inflammation Affects the Prostate on page 64.)

Noninflammatory (Category IIIb)

Also called *prostatodynia* (which literally means pain—"dynia"—in the prostate), the cause of noninflammatory prostatitis is just as mysterious as that of inflammatory prostatitis. However, unlike its inflammatory cousin Category IIIa, the prostatic secretions of men with *noninflammatory chronic abacterial prostatitis* are not swarming with inflammatory leukocytes.

Although opinions vary, most urologists agree that one or more of the following three causes can produce the symptoms of noninflammatory prostatitis:

- **Abnormal muscle spasms** of the pelvis, the external urethral striated sphincter muscle, and those that surround the bladder neck.
- **Stress** increases the release of chemicals from the involuntary nervous system, which in turn regulates contraction of smooth muscles in the bladder neck and prostate.
- **Reflux of urine into the prostate,** which can irritate prostatic tissue even if the urine is sterile. Uric acid, often present in the urine, can form crystals if the level is too high, which can cause prostatitis if they are refluxed into the prostate.

ASYMPTOMATIC INFLAMMATORY PROSTATITIS (CATEGORY IV)

By definition, men with category IV prostatitis are asymptomatic. In general, this type of prostatitis is detected incidentally when prostatic tissue is removed for other reasons—for example, when prostate tissue is removed subsequent to a prostate biopsy or following surgery for an enlarged or cancerous prostate. Less frequently, this type of prostatitis is discovered when inflammatory cells (leukocytes) are found in the prostatic secretions of asymptomatic men.

POSSIBLE COMPLICATIONS OF PROSTATITIS

The consequences of prostatitis can be significant—even life-threatening. For instance, if certain types of bacteria (*Escherichia coli,* for example) enter the bloodstream and release a toxic substance called *endotoxin,* it can be fatal. Endotoxin causes blood vessels to become leaky—they let excess fluid pour into surrounding tissue. When enough fluid leaks out, the blood pressure plummets, causing shock. Fortunately, warning signs (such as fever and chills) accompanied by urinary tract symptoms (such as painful and frequent urination) appear long before shock occurs.

However, most cases of acute bacterial prostatitis aren't life-threatening, but delayed treatment can still have serious consequences. For instance, if swarms of bacteria are allowed to proliferate, they can form an abscess. An abscess must be drained (usually by surgery) before the infection can be eliminated.

Finally, if the bacterial infection isn't completely eradicated, it sets the stage for a chronically infected prostate and recurrent urinary tract infections (since bacteria from the prostate can seep into the urine). In fact, chronic bacterial prostatitis is the leading cause of recurrent urinary tract infection in men. Just the same, using antibiotics to treat an "infection," when there isn't one, risks other adverse side effects.

Prompt diagnosis and treatment of bacterial prostatitis not only provides the best chance for a cure; it also reduces the chances of serious complications. Therefore, at the first sign of prostate infection, don't delay. See your doctor immediately or go to the nearest emergency room.

Diagnosing Prostatitis

Like other aspects of the disorder, the diagnosis of every type of prostatitis (except acute bacterial prostatitis) is controversial. In theory, most textbooks neatly classify the various types according to the presence or absence of bacteria and inflammatory cells. In clinical practice, though, the division between the different types of chronic prostatitis is fuzzy at best.

How Inflammation Affects the Prostate

Similar to how sunburn causes fluid accumulation within a blister, prostatic inflammation causes fluid accumulation within the prostate. In the case of a blister, with further fluid accumulation, the skin stretches, which allows the blister to grow in size. In the case of prostatitis, though, excess fluid doesn't have anywhere else to go—the prostate is encased within a rigid capsule of fibrous tissue. Therefore, as the prostate swells with fluid, the pressure is directed inward. Consequently, the prostate becomes squeezed tighter and tighter. Like a nutcracker, this pressure compresses the prostatic tissue, the prostatic ducts, and the nerves that innervate the prostate.

This squeezing sensation causes pain. Although the pain originates within the prostate, it can radiate elsewhere. For instance, the pain can radiate along the nerves that supply the prostate. In other words, the aching sensation of a swollen prostate isn't just confined to the prostate. The pain can be referred from the prostate to other areas deep within the pelvis, above the pubic bone, in the perineum (skin between the testicles and anus), or even into the upper thighs.

SYMPTOMS

With the exception of fever and chills (which is seen with acute bacterial prostatitis), men with other types of chronic prostatitis have similar symptoms. These symptoms include urinary symptoms (such as urgent, frequent, and painful urination) or physical complaints (such as genital, pelvic, and lower abdominal pain).

PHYSICAL EXAMINATION

The physical examination is also similar between the various categories of chronic prostatitis. Findings range from a normal prostate exam to varying degrees of swelling and tenderness. (Note: A rectal examination is not recommended in suspected acute bacterial prostatitis, because it might squeeze bacteria into the bloodstream.)

LAB TESTS

In addition to taking a detailed history and performing a thorough physical examination, urologists often perform tests on urine and prostatic secretions.

With the exception of bacterial prostatitis (categories I and II), a *urinalysis* (microscopic examination of the urine) and *urine culture* (where a sample of urine is sent to a laboratory and cultured or grown) is unremarkable. In the case of bacterial prostatitis, bacteria in the urine are often visible under the microscope, and a urine culture is usually positive (grows bacteria).

Examining *expressed prostatic secretions* (EPS) under the microscope is another way of distinguishing between the different types of prostatitis. These secretions are obtained by milking (massaging) the prostate gland during a digital rectal exam. This fluid is then examined for the presence or absence of bacteria and leukocytes. However, many urologists don't routinely examine or culture prostatic secretions before treating prostatitis. Instead, they diagnose and treat prostatitis based on the present symptoms, such as pelvic pain and difficult urination.

CONDITIONS THAT MIMIC PROSTATITIS

Since the origin of prostatitis is unknown in the majority of cases, and the diagnosis is based primarily on symptoms, treatment is often based on trial and error. One reason that the cure rate is so dismal is that a faulty diagnosis has been made. In other words, the patient is suffering from a condition other than prostatitis. Conditions that can masquerade as noninflammatory chronic prostatitis include interstitial cystitis (a disabling condition of the bladder), bladder cancer, and prostate cancer. Interstitial cystitis (IC), in particular, has similar symptoms—frequent painful urination, sexual dysfunction, and pelvic pain—so men with IC are often treated unsuccessfully for years before they are properly diagnosed. (For more information on research and current IC treatment, contact The Interstitial Cystitis Association, listed in the Resources section on page 173.)

Conventional Treatment of Prostatitis

Urologists treat prostatitis with a combination of art and science. From a practical standpoint, the *art* of treating prostatitis includes time-honored measures such as drinking plenty of water, avoiding constipation, reducing stress, and eliminating urinary irritants (such as spicy foods, alcoholic beverages, and caffeine). It also includes a trial-and-error process of using different remedies to treat the symptoms of prostatitis (often without scientific proof that the patient actually has the condition).

The *science* of treating prostatitis involves using specific therapies that are based on scientific facts—for instance, using a specific antibiotic to treat "culture-proven" bacterial prostatitis. Urologists prove that a patient has bacterial prostatitis by culturing (growing) a sample of urine or prostatic secretion in a nutrient broth. If any bacteria are present, they start to multiply and form colonies on the surface of the nutrient broth that are visible to the naked eye.

In the following pages, I'll share with you how urologists weave art with science to treat prostatitis as we explore conventional treatments.

ANTIBIOTICS

Urologists rely on antibiotics more than any other method to treat all forms of prostatitis, even though only a small percent of men have proven to have bacterial prostatitis.

Before administering antibiotics for proven bacterial prostatitis, doctors try to choose the best antibiotic for the job. Although multiple antibiotics may be effective, in some cases only a single antibiotic will work. If a patient is sick, doctors treat the infection empirically—that is, they make an educated guess based on their experience and the patient's medical history. In less serious situations, doctors often wait and choose the most appropriate antibiotic based on the results of a *culture and sensitivity report*. This report indicates if the cultured bacteria are sensitive to a particular antibiotic. Antibiotics kill bacteria by interfering with various parts of their growth cycle. If bacteria can't grow, they die. To be effective, an antibiotic must:

- penetrate the prostate
- reach the bacteria
- achieve a concentration within the prostatic tissue that is sufficient to kill the bacteria
- be taken long enough to kill all the bacteria

Unfortunately, the results of antibiotic therapies for prostatitis leave much to be desired. Without question, the biggest reason that antibiotics fail is that they're used inappropriately.

Bacterial Prostatitis

In theory, only bacterial prostatitis (the rarest type of prostatitis) should be treated with antibiotics. If there isn't an infection, antibiotics can do more harm than good. If the four criteria above are met, acute bacterial prostatitis can be cured in about three to four weeks. In contrast, the cure rate for chronic bacterial prostatitis is dismal. Even though men are treated with prolonged courses of antibiotics (ranging anywhere from months to years), the majority of them aren't permanently cured.

Chronic Abacterial Prostatitis

Although antibiotics are specific only for bacterial prostatitis, most urologists try at least one course of antibiotics for *all types* of prostatitis. Not surprisingly (since there isn't a bacterial infection), the results are often the same whether antibiotics are given or not—approximately one-third of men with chronic abacterial prostatitis (categories IIIa and IIIb) are cured, but similar results have been achieved with a placebo.

Asymptomatic Inflammatory Prostatitis

Although asymptomatic inflammatory prostatitis is usually not treated with antibiotics (since it's asymptomatic), urologists resort to antibiotic therapy under certain circumstances. These situations include cases of infertility due to pus in the semen; an elevated PSA level; or before inserting an instrument, such as a cystoscope, into the urethra and bladder.

Like my colleagues, I restrict antibiotic therapy to the situations listed above. However, in contrast to other urologists, I treat *all* men with asymptomatic inflammatory prostatitis with natural anti-inflammatory therapies. Here's why. According to a respected Johns Hopkins researcher, chronic prostatic inflammation may increase the risk of developing benign and malignant (cancerous) prostate disease because it stimulates prostate cell growth.[1]

PROSTATIC MASSAGE

Used for centuries to treat prostate problems, prostatic massage for chronic bacterial prostatitis has been making a comeback, thanks to the pioneering work of Filipino physician Antonio Feliciano and his father. These two men have improved the quality of life of thousands of men with prostatitis by combining a program of regular prostate massage—usually three times a week for four to eight weeks—with traditional treatment (such as antibiotics and dietary and lifestyle changes).

The procedure is straightforward. First, a gloved, well-lubricated index finger is carefully inserted into the rectum. Next, the outside surface of the prostate is palpated (felt). The prostate, which lies just beneath the anterior (upper) surface of the rectum, measures about the size of a golf ball; it feels like the tip of your nose. Prostatic massage forces secretions laden with dead bacteria and cellular debris into the urethra. Urination washes the secretions to the outside.

This massaging maneuver is continued progressively from the base of the prostate to the apex (anterior portion of the prostate, closest to the anus). Although this procedure is usually performed by a urologist, a motivated patient or loved one can also be taught how to perform prostate massage.

Dr. Feliciano reports that improvement usually begins after the fourth treatment. Complete relief, though, usually requires an additional six to fourteen treatments.[2] According to researchers at Stanford University School of Medicine, regular prostatic massage reduces the pain of chronic prostatitis by over 50 percent.[3]

MUSCLE RELAXATION

Although unproven, urologists believe that inflammatory and non-inflammatory chronic abacterial prostatitis is caused by spasms of the muscles that control urination. In addition, smooth muscle spasm can cause or aggravate bacterial prostatitis by causing urinary reflux into the prostate.

To alleviate muscle spasms, urologists often prescribe an anti-anxiety medication called Valium (benzodiazepam) to promote muscle relaxation and reduce stress. They also prescribe drugs that are primarily used to treat an enlarged prostate, called alpha-adrenergic blockers. Alpha-blockers work by relaxing smooth muscle in the prostate and bladder neck (see page 39). Although one-third of patients are cured, two-thirds still complain of their symptoms.

Physical Therapy

According to researchers at the Cleveland Clinic, tailor-made physical therapy that targets specific muscles in the pelvis and back can alleviate prostatitis symptoms. Of the twenty-one men who completed a prescribed exercise program, fifteen (71 percent) experienced a greater than 50 percent improvement in their prostatitis symptoms.[4]

Muscle relaxation is best achieved with natural methods, such as biofeedback training and muscle relaxation exercises. (See page 79.)

ANTI-INFLAMMATORY MEDICATIONS

An acutely infected prostate is markedly swollen and inflamed. Although less dramatic than the acute version, a chronically infected prostate is also inflamed.

Finally, even though the cause is unknown, chronic inflammatory abacterial prostatitis is characterized by the presence of inflammatory cells. Perhaps this explains why most urologists prescribe anti-inflammatory medications (such as ibuprofen) for prostatitis. Finasteride, a prescription medication that is used to treat prostate enlargement (see page 40), can also decrease prostatic inflammation.

Although anti-inflammatory medications can't cure prostatitis, they can reduce prostatic inflammation. Regardless of the mechanism, as far as the patient is concerned, the only thing that matters is the relief of symptoms. Anti-inflammatory medications help approximately one-third of men with prostatitis.

TRANSURETHRAL MICROWAVE THERAPY

According to Canadian researchers, transurethral microwave therapy (see page 44) is an effective, safe, and durable treatment for nonbacterial prostatitis that is unresponsive to traditional therapies.[5] These researchers divided twenty men with nonbacterial prostatitis into two groups. One group was treated with microwave therapy, and the other group was treated with a placebo treatment. At three months following therapy, all of the men in the treatment group, versus none of the men in the sham group, experienced an improvement in their voiding symptoms and quality of life. After twenty-one months, 70 percent of the men in the treatment group still experienced improvement.

PSYCHOLOGICAL COUNSELING

Chronic prostatitis exacts a heavy emotional toll on men. To begin with, men with chronic prostatitis are usually depressed. They're plagued with persistent pelvic, prostatic, and genital pain; difficult, frequent, and painful urination; impaired fertility; and diminished sexual performance. These factors conspire to sap the joy from everyday living. To add insult to injury, these men also have to contend with unrewarding doctor visits, innumerable laboratory tests, and countless medications. Finally, the emotional fallout from their battle with chronic prostatitis adversely affects their family members and coworkers.

Psychological counseling can help alleviate the pain and suffering that accompany chronic prostatitis by providing men with new coping skills (such as stress-management techniques). Counseling also can facilitate the grieving process that accompanies any chronic illness.

Natural Remedies for Prostatitis

Shortly after I began practicing urology, I became frustrated with what modern medicine had to offer for treating prostatitis. Accepting this as a challenge, I began a quest for natural alternatives. Although my quest is far from being over, I've discovered a treasure trove of natural remedies for prostatitis and a variety of other conditions as you'll see below.

Natural remedies for prostatitis can be divided into two broad categories—general and specific remedies. General remedies, like the ones discussed here through page 82 can be used for every type of prostatitis. Specific remedies, which begin on page 82 with the section "Herbal Remedies," are used to treat a specific complaint or symptom, such as burning during urination. For successful treatment, both types should be used.

Lifestyle—daily choices that are under our control—can either improve or worsen the symptoms of prostatitis. Healthy choices (such as exercising regularly, getting enough rest, and reducing stress) improve these symptoms and contribute to your overall health and happiness.

REDUCE STRESS

While stress is a part of everyday life, heightened levels of stress worsen the symptoms of prostatitis. Prolonged stress increases the incidence of urinary tract infections, depresses the immune system, and increases spasms of the bladder, urethral, and pelvic musculature. Although stress can't be eliminated, it can be controlled with the following techniques.

Exercise

Prolonged sitting increases the risk of developing prostatitis. Regular exercise is a great way to reduce stress and the symptoms of prostatitis. As an added bonus, regular exercise improves immune function; promotes normal sleep; prevents depression; lowers blood pressure and serum cholesterol; reduces the risk of osteoporosis; assists with weight loss; and averts many types of cancer (including prostate cancer). Adjust your schedule so you can exercise before or after work. Find an exercise that you enjoy. Develop a program that includes a balance of aerobic exercise (walking, running, biking, swimming), and resistance training such as weight lifting. (Note: If you're a bicycle enthusiast, be aware that bikes with narrow seats increase the risk of prostatitis [and impotence] by compressing the prostate and the pudendal nerve, which controls erections. Therefore, select a well-padded seat that is designed to minimize pressure on the perineum [area between the scrotum and anus.]) *Be sure to consult with your physician before embarking on a new exercise program.*

Meditate

Meditation is a form of mental relaxation, a form of contemplation. There are many meditation techniques to choose from. Experiment and pick a technique that feels comfortable to you. If you need help getting started, join a meditation class, attend a retreat, buy a self-help book, or purchase an instructional audiotape on meditation (they're available in most bookstores).

Practice Deep Breathing

Begin by placing your hand on your belly. Take a deep breath and cause your hand to rise first. Continue drawing the rest of the breath into your lungs, from the bottom up. Pause, then reverse the process. Finish by depressing your diaphragm to expel the last bit of air from your lungs. Pause. Then start over again. Reduce stress by practicing diaphragmatic breathing frequently throughout the day.

Avoid Violent Movies, Books, and Music

Violence in any form increases stress by jarring the emotions. Violence revs up the immune system by causing the adrenal glands to release adrenaline (the "fight-or-flight" hormone). Repeated jump-starting of the immune system causes unnecessary wear and tear, which depresses immune function.

Practice Yoga

Originating in the Far East, yoga is an ancient tradition that combines stretching and breathing exercises with meditation. Having practiced yoga for years, I can attest to its benefits. I routinely recommend it to my patients. There are many excellent books on the subject, and because yoga has become so popular, the chances are good that classes are available in your neighborhood. Try your local fitness center first.

Get Enough Sleep
Try to get at least seven hours of sleep daily. Relaxing sleep improves immune function, reduces depression, prevents fatigue, and enhances pain tolerance.

Practice Forgiveness
Of all the lessons I've learned over the years, perhaps the most valuable is the healing power of forgiveness. I've come to understand that forgiveness is a gift we give ourselves. It sets us free. I've observed that patients who learn to forgive and love themselves and others are happier and healthier people.

Take Time to Smell the Roses
Although life can be a rat race, it doesn't have to be. The choice is yours. Become an expert at living. Live each day to the fullest and discover its many miracles.

Try Bach Flower Essences
Dr. Edward Bach, an English medical doctor and homeopathic physician, discovered that flower essences could reduce stress and a number of other ailments. Dr. Bach discovered that every flower has its own unique healing properties. By using a process of trial and error, he uncovered the healing qualities of thirty-eight different flower essences. Bach flower essences are available in most health food stores. I recommend trying a combination of five different Bach flower essences called rescue formula. Apply four drops under the tongue whenever you're under stress. I've taken it. It works.

ELIMINATE TOBACCO, ALCOHOL, AND CAFFEINE
Breakdown products of tobacco, alcohol, and caffeine-containing foods or beverages irritate the prostate and aggravate the symptoms of prostatitis.

(Smoking tobacco and drinking alcohol also increase the risk of prostate cancer.) Avoid them.

DRINK PLENTY OF WATER

Water dilutes noxious chemicals found in urine. Concentrated urine irritates the bladder and prostate; diluted urine soothes them. Drink enough water to make at least two quarts of urine daily—at least eight 8-ounce glasses of water every twenty-four hours. Drinking sufficient water also prevents constipation—another problem that aggravates prostate problems.

DIET

Although usually taken for granted, food is a potent medicine. Like a drug, the ingredients contained within food have a profound influence on the body. Protein molecules embedded within certain foods (such as wheat and sugar) can induce a migraine headache, exacerbate arthritis, provoke a diffuse skin rash, or even aggravate the symptoms of prostatitis.

Avoid Hot, Spicy Foods

The ingredients found in hot spicy foods are excreted in the urine. These foods irritate an inflamed prostate. Avoid them if you have prostatitis.

Avoid Refined Sugar

Sugar depresses the immune system by preventing white blood cells from doing their job—engulfing bacteria. In place of refined sugar, use the herbal sweetener stevia *(Stevia rebaudiana)*. Available in most health food stores, stevia contains only one-tenth of a calorie per teaspoon.

Reduce Fat

Inflammation aggravates prostatitis symptoms, so it makes sense to avoid foods that promote it, such as fat. In particular, avoid foods that contain saturated fat (animal fat)—the type of fat in junk food, meat, and dairy products.

Avoid Foods That Increase Uric Acid

Uric acid, a by-product of purine metabolism, is excreted in the urine. If the uric acid level in the urine is too high (determined by a simple urine test), uric acid crystals start to form. Reflux of uric acid crystals into the prostate can cause irritation and inflammation. Limit foods high in purine, such as meat and seafood, and drink enough extra fluid to produce two to three quarts of urine daily. Also, drink fresh lemonade made with real lemon juice and sweetened with stevia, not refined sugar. Lemon juice alkalinizes urine.

Avoid Foods That Cause an Allergic Reaction

Food allergies can cause prostatitis symptoms. Men with food allergies are usually unaware that foods (usually the ones they crave) may be causing their symptoms. Eliminating problem foods can alleviate prostatitis symptoms. Experiment by following a "food elimination diet" for three weeks (see page 77).

Eat Foods That Reduce Inflammation

Certain foods decrease or relieve the symptoms of prostatitis by reducing inflammation. Increased oxidant damage within the prostate (caused by infection and inflammation) provokes the symptoms of prostatitis. Fresh fruits and vegetables (particularly the bright-colored ones, such as yellow squash, carrots, and blueberries) are a rich source of antioxidant vitamins and minerals. Antioxidant vitamins soothe the inflammatory changes caused by prostatitis. Eat at least five servings of fresh fruits and vegetables daily.

Foods rich in soy protein (such as tofu, tempeh, and soy milk) dramatically decrease the incidence of prostatitis, at least in rats.[6] Eat at least two daily servings of soy protein, or take a supplement of genistein. (See page 134, for more information on soy protein.)

An anti-inflammatory molecule called prostaglandin E3 is derived from omega-3 essential fatty acids contained in flaxseed. Flaxseeds are also packed with a nutritious fiber called lignan, which helps alleviate constipation, a potential cause of prostatitis. It is also a rich source of phytoestrogens, which prevent prostate cancer. I recommend using defatted flaxseed meal, which is available in most health food stores.

Food Elimination Diet[7]

Foods that induce an allergic reaction in the body can cause or exacerbate prostatitis-like symptoms. Fortunately, the remedy is simple: adhere to the following food elimination diet for three weeks.

- **Restricted foods.** Eliminate immediately the following common food allergens: dairy products, wheat, corn, eggs, citrus fruits, coffee, tea, alcohol, refined sugar, food additives, and any other food you eat more than three times a week. Also, eliminate any known food allergens. Read food labels. Packaged foods contain many of these foods.
- **Allowed foods.** Don't worry, you won't starve. You can still eat the following foods: cereals, grains (except wheat and corn), legumes (beans), fresh vegetables, poultry, fowl, fresh fish, nuts (except peanuts), seeds, soy milk, and herbal teas.
- **Food challenge test.** Once the three weeks have passed, introduce one restricted food each day. Test pure sources of a food. For instance, for wheat, use a pure wheat cereal without milk, corn, sugar, or other additives. Eat a sizable portion of the test food at each meal. Keep a food diary and record any adverse reactions. Allergic reactions usually appear within ten minutes to twelve hours after ingesting the test food, but they can take as long as three to four days to manifest. If symptoms develop, avoid the food. Wait until the symptoms completely disappear before testing another food. Eliminate foods that cause an allergic reaction. Vary the remaining "safe foods" by rotating the types of food you eat each day.
- **Other benefits.** As a bonus, a food elimination diet may improve other chronic health problems that have been linked to food allergies. These include depression, sinusitis, irritable bowel syndrome, constipation, rheumatoid arthritis, headaches, and asthma.

SITZ BATHS

The word *sitz* means "to sit or soak your pelvis in a tub of water." A traditional European folk remedy, a soothing sitz bath usually provides immediate comfort to an aching prostate. You can take a hot or cold one, or a combination of both called a *contrast sitz bath*.

Taking a hot sitz bath for fifteen minutes twice daily improves the symptoms of prostatitis. The water should be hot but not scalding. Hot water improves immune function by stimulating the swallowing of bacteria by white cells and by reducing stress. A hot sitz bath also increases blood flow to the prostate, thereby reducing prostatic inflammation.

A cold sitz bath reduces inflammation. A contrast sitz bath is performed by alternating a warm and cold sitz bath in the following manner:

- Fill a tub or basin with hot water (about 110° F.) so that it covers your pelvis.
- Prepare a basin of ice water and position it next to the basin or tub.
- Sit in the warm sitz bath for three to four minutes.
- Sit in the ice-water basin for thirty to sixty seconds. (Brrrrr!)
- Or place a small towel in the ice-water basin next to the tub. Then carefully kneel in the hot water (being careful not to slip). Draw the cold towel between your legs, over the pelvis, from the front to the back. Hold the towel in place for thirty to sixty seconds.
- Finally, resume sitting in the hot sitz bath.
- Repeat this routine three to five times. End with the cold-water treatment.

(**Caution:** *Sitting in a tub of hot water can make you light-headed. Therefore, come to a kneeling position and get your bearings before standing to get out of the tub.*)

Certain herbs (for instance, yarrow and ginger) decrease inflammation. Try adding a ginger and yarrow herbal infusion (tea) to a hot sitz bath. Adding essential oils to hot sitz bathwater can also decrease inflammation and reduce stress. Try adding five drops of lavender oil to your bathwater. Consult a book on aromatherapy and experiment with other essential oils that reduce stress. Use caution, though, since certain essential oils (such as cinnamon) can cause a skin reaction if applied directly to the skin. Another option is to use an atomizer, a device that emits a fine mist of essential oil into the air.

Finally, as part of your sitz bath routine, practice the "Healing Imagery for the Prostate" exercise in the inset on page 83. Healing imagery can make your prostatitis symptoms evaporate into thin air. Be creative. Play soothing music and light some candles. Relax and enjoy the experience.

MUSCLE RELAXATION EXERCISES

Spasms of the pelvic musculature—particularly the levator ani muscles (a group of muscles that surrounds the rectum and prostate) and muscles that control urination (the bladder neck and external urethral striated sphincter musculature)—increase the incidence and symptoms of prostatitis. Reduce prostatitis symptoms by trying the following:

Biofeedback Training

Biofeedback training is a method of learning how to consciously control normally unconscious bodily functions (such as heart rate, breathing, and blood pressure). Two of the muscle groups that contribute to the symptoms of prostatitis (the levator ani and bladder neck muscles) fall into this category. Biofeedback training can bring these muscles under our conscious control. It also can be used to reduce or eliminate spasms of muscles that are already under our conscious control—for instance, the external urethral striated sphincter muscle. (More information on biofeedback training is available in the "Resources" section on page 167.)

Progressive Muscle Relaxation Exercise

Progressively contracting, then relaxing, voluntary muscles throughout the body can be used to decrease tension in the muscles that control urination. Try the progressive muscle relaxation exercise in the inset on page 80. You may find it helpful to record the instructions on tape, then listen to them as you perform the exercises.

REGULAR SEXUAL ACTIVITY

"Regular" sexual activity means what's regular for you. Too little sex causes congestion—prostate secretions build up, causing the prostate to become swollen. On the other hand, too much sex—particularly if it's not your normal routine—can irritate the prostate. Find a happy medium.

Progressive Muscle Relaxation Exercise

Muscle spasms can cause or provoke prostatitis. Soothe your prostate and give the rest of your body a break by practicing the following relaxation exercise at least once daily and any time prostatitis symptoms flare.

- First, focus your attention on your hands. Make a tight fist, clenching your hands as tightly as you can. Feel the tension. Hold it for five seconds, then relax. Notice the difference.
- Next, flex your arm as tightly as you can. Hold it for five seconds, then relax. Notice the difference.
- Continue progressively contracting, then relaxing, the muscles in your forehead, jaw, neck, and shoulders.
- Then move to your lungs. Take a deep breath. Hold it as long as you can. Feel the pressure in the muscles between your ribs. When you're ready, exhale. Notice the difference.
- Now tense the muscles in your buttocks and upper thighs. Hold for five seconds, then relax. Spasms of these muscles can exacerbate the symptoms of prostatitis. Learn to relax them.
- Next, draw your toes upward, tensing your shins. Hold for five seconds, then relax.
- Then flex your toes, stretching your calf muscles. Hold for five seconds, then relax.
- Finally, notice how your muscles feel warm and relaxed, free of tension. (Pause for a minute or so.)

Regular sexual activity reduces stress. Sharing sexual intimacy also improves the quality of life for you and your partner. Partners of men suffering with prostatitis often feel shunned. Fearing they may transmit an infection to their partner (they won't), men with chronic prostatitis often avoid sexual relations altogether. Men also avoid sexual activity because of pain they experience during or after an orgasm. Fortunately, learning to relax the pelvic muscles and taking selected herbs can decrease or eliminate painful orgasms. However, don't engage in sexual activity during an acute infection.

MENTAL CONDITIONING

I've often wondered why some patients heal more quickly than others with the same condition (such as prostatitis). I believe the answer can be traced to differences in their mental attitude and coping skills. Men with healthy coping skills heal faster. They have more flexibility, a sense of control, and a positive, take-charge attitude. Their immune systems are more resilient.

What we think and say influence the health and healing of every cell in our bodies. The spoken word embodies sound energy. It bridges the inner subjective and the outer objective world. It makes manifest our inner thoughts. Our thoughts are an inner dialogue we have with ourselves. They form the dominant energies we communicate to our bodies. Hence, the healing or destructive power of the mind upon the body profoundly influences the quality of life for men suffering with prostatitis.

Practice healing speech and thoughts. Start on the road to recovery by practicing the following:

- **Learn all you can about your condition.** Become informed by doing your homework. Learn all you can about prostatitis. Quit thinking of yourself as a victim. Quit asking "Why me?"
- **Ask, "What is my body trying to tell me?"** Symptoms— sensations we feel (such as pain or a burning sensation)— are the language our bodies use to get our attention. Your body is telling you something, and you need to listen.
- **Think positive.** Stop negative self-talk. Replace negative statements such as "I'll never get rid of this prostatitis" with positive affirmations. For instance, repeat the following affirmation to yourself silently or verbally: "Every day, in every way, I'm getting better and better. My prostate is getting healthier and healthier. My prostatitis is gone." Repeat these and other healing statements that have special meaning to you. Jot them down on a piece of paper, and any time a negative thought surfaces, or your prostatitis symptoms start to flare, replace negative thoughts or feelings of despair with positive

affirmations. You'll be surprised at how quickly your body learns how to respond to your new, healthier dialogue.

- **Pray.** Finally, prayer—a means of communicating our inner thoughts with the Divine—can have a positive effect on prostatitis. I routinely use prayer in my practice of medicine. I've discovered that prayer is an integral part of the healing process. I encourage men to pray for a healthy prostate.

IMAGERY

Imagery is a form of mental shorthand, a language we use to communicate with our bodies. Images—our conscious and unconscious thoughts—are constantly being transmitted to every cell of our bodies. Healthy images (such as hope, positive anticipation, and love) promote healing. Unhealthy images (such as fear, negative anticipation, and hate) have the opposite effect.

Although it may seem foreign at first, mastering mental imagery is not as difficult as you might imagine. With practice, you can learn to send healing messages to your prostate.

Use the breathing exercise on page 83 to compose a healing message to your prostate that can improve, or even eliminate, the nagging symptoms of prostatitis. You may also want to combine this exercise with the muscle relaxation exercise described on page 80. Deep breathing decreases smooth muscle spasms by decreasing stress and decreasing stimulation from the sympathetic nervous system.

In addition to this deep breathing exercise, I encourage you to seek additional resources on guided imagery, which can help form a positive, healthy image. These resources are listed on page 169.

Herbal Remedies

I routinely recommend herbal remedies to men with prostatitis. Although herbs work more slowly than prescription drugs (it can take four to six weeks to achieve maximum improvement), herbs cost less and cause fewer side effects. Furthermore, herbal remedies generally alleviate the

Healing Imagery for the Prostate

To engage in healing imagery, find a comfortable spot where you won't be disturbed. You may wish to play some soft meditative music. Keeping your eyelids shut will minimize distractions. Sit with your spine straight, centered over your pelvis, your hands folded in your lap, your feet placed flat on the floor. Alternatively, you can lie flat on your back (but don't fall asleep). You may wish to record the entire exercise on an audiotape. Give yourself plenty of time between steps to visualize each one. Then you can listen to the recording with earphones every time you practice this exercise.

- Begin by breathing naturally through your nose. Notice how the air passes gently through your nostrils. Feel your belly rise and fall as you breathe in and out.
- When you're ready, take a deep breath. Feel your belly rise first. Then, as you continue to inhale, draw the breath into your lungs from the bottom up. Feel your chest expand. Pause. Notice the sensation.
- When you're ready, reverse the process. Exhale and force the air from your lungs by compressing your diaphragm. Feel the rush of air as it passes through gently pursed lips. Pause. Notice the sensation.
- Then begin again. Inhale and exhale several more times. Feel more relaxed with each inhalation. As you exhale, feel any tension float away. Continue breathing gently for another minute or so.
- Now imagine that your breath is a colorful, healing mist (your choice of colors). As you inhale, visualize this luminous vapor filling your lungs. Notice how your red cells become illuminated as they stream through the lungs. See them shimmer and glow as they float to every part of your body.
- Watch as billions of gleaming red cells infuse their healing glow into every cell in your body. In particular, notice how the cells within your prostate become immersed in scintillating healing light. Feel the nurturing healing energy. Experience a soothing sensation radiating throughout your prostate.
- As healing light energy floods into your prostate, observe how "dark" energies (such as inflammation, infection, and pain) are carried away by the red cells as they make their way back to the lungs.

(continued)

- In the lungs, notice how the red cells release their packets of dark energy in exchange for packets of healing light energy. Then watch as the dark energies float away with each exhalation. Feel the nagging symptoms of prostatitis disappear. Feel a sense of relief flowing throughout your body. Pause.
- Repeat the breathing exercise several more times. When you're finished, picture a perfectly healthy prostate pulsating with vibrant healing light. (Pause for a minute or so.)
- In your mind's eye, picture one of your favorite places, perhaps a spot in the forest or by a lake—a healing place. Take your time and draw upon all five senses to make your image as real as possible.
- When you're ready, silently repeat the positive healing affirmations listed on page 81, or others that have special meaning for you, such as "My prostate is now free of infection. My prostate is now free of pain. My prostate is free of inflammation. My prostate is now perfectly healthy."

symptoms of prostatitis (especially nonbacterial prostatitis) more effectively than do prescription medications.

For your convenience, I have organized this section according to the symptoms of prostatitis and the herbal remedies that alleviate them. (**Note:** Herbs can be taken either singly or in combination. If improvement hasn't occurred within four to six weeks, try a different herbal combination.)

HERBS THAT DECREASE SWELLING AND INFLAMMATION

Fortunately, painful prostatitis symptoms that are caused by swelling and inflammation can be treated naturally. These symptoms can be improved by taking the following herbs, either singly or in combination.

Saw Palmetto Berry *(Serenoa repens)*

As discussed in Chapter 2, saw palmetto reduces inflammation and swelling in the prostate. Researchers treated one group of men with saw palmetto for twelve weeks prior to an open prostatectomy, a procedure in which only the inside of the prostate gland is removed. Another group of men was given a placebo (sugar pill). When the excised prostate tissue was compared under the microscope, there was significantly less prostatic swelling and inflammation in the saw palmetto group as compared to the placebo group.[8]

The recommended daily dose is 160 milligrams of a fat-soluble extract (standardized to contain 85 to 95 percent fatty acids and sterols), taken twice daily for men weighing less than 200 pounds, and three times daily for men over 200 pounds. Although it is often recommended that you take the daily amount of saw palmetto in divided doses, it also appears to work just as well if the entire dose is taken once daily. There are no contraindications, known drug interactions, or significant side effects other than occasional stomach upset. (See page 50 for more information.)

Pygeum *(Prunus africana)*

Although pygeum has been used by European physicians for decades (and by African natives for millennia) to treat prostate enlargement and prostatitis, it is virtually unknown to most American physicians. Native to Africa, the bark of the tree is harvested, then ground into a fine powder for medicinal purposes.

Like saw palmetto, pygeum prevents inflammatory changes within the prostate by blocking the conversion of arachidonic acid to its inflammatory by-products. Similarly, it decreases edema (fluid collection) within the prostate.

I recommend taking a standardized, lipophilic (fat-soluble) extract of pygeum that contains 14 percent triterpenes and a half percent *n*-docosanol. Take 100 to 200 milligrams daily in divided doses (if used in combination with other herbs, use the lower dosage). There are no contraindications, drug interactions, or serious side effects, except occasional nausea and stomach pains. (See page 52 for more information.)

Cernilton

This patented pollen-derived product was first formulated in Sweden more than fifty years ago. Nevertheless, most American urologists have never heard of it. That's unfortunate, because Cernilton has been used worldwide to successfully treat BPH (see page 54) and nonbacterial prostatitis.

It is one of the most promising herbal treatments I've come across to treat prostatitis. In fact, I've had such good results from using Cernilton that it's now my first-line treatment for prostatitis.

Among other things, Cernilton contains vitamins, minerals, amino acids, and phytosterols. Also found in many of the other herbs that are used to treat prostatitis, phytosterols reduce edema and inflammation within the prostate by blocking the formation of inflammatory prostaglandin and leucotriene molecules.

I routinely treat men with type IV prostatitis (asymptomatic prostatitis detected on prostate biopsy) with a six-month course of Cernilton instead of antibiotics. I've been pleased with the results. I've observed that most men experience a modest improvement in their PSA blood test. In some men, the results have been even more dramatic—after taking six months of Cernilton, their PSA level has dropped by as much as 50 percent.

According to scientific research, Cernilton significantly improves the symptoms of nonbacterial prostatitis in the majority of cases (78 percent).[9] That has been my experience as well.

Cernilton is commercially available (http://www.abcernelle.com/products.html, and www.cernitinamerica.com). Take as directed on the package insert. If you're allergic to plant pollen, check with your physician before using.

South African Star Grass *(Hypoxis rooperi)*

This herbal product (brand name Harzol) is widely used throughout Europe to treat prostate problems. Derived from the roots of the South African star grass, Harzol is rich in phytosterols—a class of compounds that are related to cholesterol. Although the exact mechanism is unknown, the phytosterols (especially beta-sitosterol) are believed to reduce edema and inflammation within the prostate by inhibiting the formation of inflammatory prostaglandins.

While Harzol isn't available in this country, other beta-sitosterol-containing products are available in health food stores or by mail order (Beachwood Canyon Naturally, 888-803-5333). Select a product that contains at least 50 percent beta-sitosterol. Follow the instructions on the package. There are no serious side effects from taking the medication.

Clivers *(Galium aparine)*

Useful for prostatitis, clivers is a non-irritating diuretic herb that reduces irritation and inflammation within the prostate. Although the exact mechanism is unknown, clivers is rich in antioxidant compounds called flavonoids. Flavonoids combat oxidative damage caused by free radicals, which induce inflammation within the prostate. Clivers is available as a fluid extract. Drink thirty to forty drops in water three times daily.

Agrimony *(Agrimonia eupatorium)*

The flowering portion of this herb is dried, then prepared as a fluid extract. Agrimony reduces inflammation within the urinary tract (including the prostate). Agrimony contains powerful antioxidants, called catechins, which cool off prostatic inflammation. Drink twenty to thirty drops in water three times a day. When agrimony is taken as directed, there are no serious side effects or health hazards.

Stinging Nettle *(Urtica dioica)*

As a young man, I vividly remember my first encounter with stinging nettle. Taking a shortcut, I wandered off a path and stumbled into a patch of stinging nettle. I didn't notice the tiny hairs that projected from their stems and leaves, but I sure felt them. Like tiny hypodermic needles, these quills injected an irritating substance up and down my bare legs, which prompted an unplanned swim in a nearby creek.

I have since discovered the friendlier side—the healing side—of stinging nettle. I now routinely prescribe stinging nettle root, which is used extensively throughout Europe for a variety of prostate conditions.

Of the over fifty compounds found in stinging nettle, polysaccharides are probably the most important. Polysaccharides—a special type of carbohydrate (sugar)—reduce inflammation and edema within the prostate by blocking the formation of inflammatory prostaglandin molecules and leukotrienes.

The normal daily dose is three to six grams, taken as a tablet or capsule containing 600 to 1,200 milligrams of a 5:1 dry extract (equivalent to three to six grams of dried nettle root), or 120 milligrams twice daily of a 10:1 extract (standardized for amino acid content). When nettle root is taken as directed, there are no significant side effects or contraindications. (Note: People who are allergic to stinging nettle should not use an unprocessed [fresh] herbal preparation. In addition, stinging nettle can occasionally cause mild stomach upset.) (See page 55 for more information.)

HERBS THAT REDUCE PAINFUL URINATION

Inflammatory changes within the bladder, prostate, or urethra cause a burning sensation during urination called *dysuria*. Drinking sufficient water (at least two quarts of water daily) and avoiding irritants such as caffeinated beverages, spicy foods, alcohol, and tobacco products can take the sting out of dysuria. Herbal therapies can also soothe painful urination. Herbs that reduce dysuria include all the herbs listed above that decrease swelling and inflammation, plus the herbs listed below. These herbs can be taken either singly or in combination. (Note: Herbs that decrease dysuria can also decrease painful ejaculation.)

Marshmallow Root *(Althaea officinalis)*

Not to be confused with the puffy white candy that you roasted on a stick over a campfire, marshmallow is an herb. Herbal products that are made from the root of this medicinal herb soothe inflamed mucous membranes, including an inflamed prostatic urethra.

Marshmallow root is available as either a tea, a liquid tincture, or a capsule. Drink several cups of tea daily, drink thirty to forty drops of liquid extract in water daily, or take capsules containing an equivalent of six grams of powdered root daily in divided doses.

Marshmallow root has no known contraindications, drug interactions, or side effects. (However, the absorption of other drugs taken simultaneously with marshmallow root may be delayed.)

Eryngo *(Eryngium campestre)*
Used to treat prostatitis and an inflamed urinary tract, the dried leaves, flowers, and roots of eryngo are used to make a tea or liquid tincture. To make a tea, add one level teaspoon of dried (ground) root in a tea caddy to a cup of boiling water. Drink three to four cups of tea daily. Also available as a tincture; drink fifty to sixty drops in water three to four times daily. Eryngo is safe when taken as directed.

Corn Silk *(Zea mays)*
Corn silk also soothes painful urination. Made from the silky strands that protrude out of the top of corn husks, corn silk is available as a dried herb (take four to eight grams of dried herb three times daily); tea (add one-half gram [about two teaspoons] of dried herb in a tea caddy to five ounces of boiling water, and drink several cups daily); or liquid tincture 1:5 in 25 percent alcohol (drink 5 to 15 milliliters—one to three teaspoons—in water three times daily). When taken as directed, corn silk is safe.

HERBS THAT INCREASE URINARY FLOW

Herbs that increase urinary output are called diuretics. The following herbs dilute noxious irritants in the urine and soothe the urinary tract by "flushing" the kidneys.

Couch Grass *(Elymus repens)*
The root of this medicinal herb increases urinary output. Available either as a tea (add three grams of ground root in a tea caddy to a cup of boiling water, and drink two to three cups daily) or as a liquid tincture (drink thirty to forty drops in water three times daily). Couch grass is safe when taken as directed.

Dandelion *(Taraxacum officinale)*
Dandelions are famous as bothersome weeds, but they are also a gentle diuretic. The root and aerial (part above ground) portion of the dandelion plant is used to make a tea (add one teaspoon of ground herb in a tea

caddy to a cup of boiling water twice daily); a tincture (drink ten to fifteen drops in water three times daily); or capsules of dried, ground herb (4:1 extract, take one capsule three times daily). In addition to being a diuretic, fresh dandelion leaves add a stimulating bitter taste to salads. "Bitters" improve digestion by stimulating bile secretion. Taken as directed, dandelion is safe (except in cases of intestinal or gallbladder obstruction).

HERBS THAT PREVENT URINARY TRACT INFECTIONS

While antibiotics are traditionally used to treat bacterial urinary tract infections (UTIs), herbal remedies can complement antibiotic therapies. For instance, certain herbs are urinary antiseptics (they sterilize the urine); others prevent recurrent urinary tract infections; still others make antibiotics work better.

Although herbal therapies aren't able to penetrate the prostate like antibiotics, they can reduce the incidence and recurrence of bacterial prostatitis by preventing urinary tract infections. (If infected urine refluxes into the prostate, it can cause bacterial prostatitis.) The herbs listed below decrease the incidence and recurrence of urinary tract infections.

Cranberry (*Vaccinium macrocarpon*)

Used as a folk remedy for centuries, there is now solid scientific evidence that cranberries can prevent recurrent bacterial UTIs. Substances that are concentrated in cranberries (called *proanthocyanidins*) prevent certain bacteria (*Escherichia coli, Proteus* spp., and *Pseudomonas aeruginosa*) from adhering to the inner lining of the bladder.[10] *Escherichia coli* causes 80 percent of the cases of bacterial prostatitis.

Cranberry juice is frequently used to prevent recurrent UTIs. Unfortunately, most commercial cranberry juices contain only one-quarter fruit—the rest of the juice is loaded with sugar (in the form of corn syrup). Therefore, select an unsweetened variety and drink eight ounces daily. Another option is to take one standardized cranberry capsule three times daily for prevention, and two capsules three times daily if infection is present. Cranberry juice and capsules are safe when taken as directed.

Uva Ursi *(Arctostaphylos uvae ursi)*

Uva ursi has pea-sized fruit that bears love, which explains why uva ursi is also called bearberry. Uva ursi is a urinary antiseptic. Arbutin, a chemical found in the leaves of uva ursi, inhibits a variety of bacteria that cause prostatitis.

Uva ursi is available as a tea (add three grams of ground herb in a tea caddy to five ounces of boiling water and drink one cup four times daily); a solid extract (the hydroquinone derivative, calculated as water-free arbutin, is dosed at 100 to 210 milligrams up to four times daily); and as a 1:1 fluid extract (drink 1.5 to 4 milliliters in water three times daily). Uva ursi is safe when taken as directed. Avoid medications or foods that acidify the urine (cranberries, for example) while taking uva ursi, since it works best in alkaline urine.

(Note: Uva ursi should not be taken for more than a week, and it's contraindicated in pregnant women, patients with renal disease, nursing mothers, and children under the age of twelve.)

Purple Coneflower *(Echinacea purpurae)*

This herb is rich in antioxidant substances (polysaccharides and flavonoids) that reduce inflammation, stimulate the immune system, and improve the ability of white cells to swallow bacteria. Other substances found in echinacea *(echinacoside* and *caffeic acid)* kill a variety of bacteria, including *Proteus vulgaris* and *Staphylococcus aureus.*

Available as a tea (add one to two grams of powdered herb in a tea caddy to boiling water, and drink one cup three times daily); standardized fluid extract (drink thirty to sixty drops in water three times daily); or solid extract (take 100 to 250 milligrams capsules containing 3.5 percent echinacoside three times daily). Although there are theoretical concerns about taking echinacea in patients with progressive systemic diseases (such as multiple sclerosis), or with immune disorders (such as AIDS), when taken orally as directed, echinacea is safe.[11]

Pipsissewa *(Chimaphila umbellata)*

This herb grows extensively in Europe, Asia, Siberia, and North and South America. The leaves from this perennial semi-shrub possess antimicrobial properties. Similar to uva ursi, pipsissewa has arbutin-containing compounds that are converted in alkaline urine to hydroquinone derivatives.

Pipsissewa is available as a powder (take capsules containing two grams of herb once daily); a tea (add one to three grams of herb to a cup of boiling once daily); or as a liquid extract (drink one to four milliliters in water once daily). The same precautions that apply for uva ursi also apply for pipsissewa.

Oregon Grape *(Mahonia aquifolium)*

Popularly known as barberry, the root of Oregon grape was used by American Indians as a tonic. A favorite of herbalists, Oregon grape is used as an "herbal antibiotic." Two constituents of Oregon grape, *berberine* and *oxyacanthine,* possess antimicrobial activity.

Oregon grape is available as a tincture (drink two to four milliliters in water three times daily) or as a powder (take one-half to one gram three times daily). Oregon grape is safe when taken as directed.

HERBS THAT MAKE ANTIBIOTICS MORE EFFECTIVE

In order to be effective, an antibiotic must achieve a concentration within the prostate that is high enough to kill any bacteria. Bromelain, a group of enzymes derived from pineapple *(Ananas comusus)*, increases the concentration of penicillin and tetracycline—two antibiotics that are frequently used to treat prostatitis—within the urine and the cells that line the prostatic ducts. Bromelain also improves the absorption of quercetin (see page 96), an antioxidant supplement that reduces prostatitis symptoms.

Commercially available bromelain is derived from the stem, not the fruit, of the pineapple plant. The dosage depends on the preparation. The activity of bromelain is expressed in an enzyme unit called a *milk clotting unit* (mcu). The typical dose of bromelain is 250 to 500 milligrams (of a product containing between 1,200 and 1,800 mcu) taken three times daily between meals. When taken as directed, bromelain is safe. (**Note:** Bromelain is contraindicated in cases of hypersensitivity to bromelain [pineapple]. Also, avoid taking bromelain along with blood thinners.)

HERBS THAT REDUCE STRESS AND MUSCLE SPASMS

As pointed out earlier, stress and muscle spasms can increase the incidence of prostatitis. Prescription medications, such as benzodiazepines (Valium, for example), are addictive, impair mental function, and cause drowsiness. Natural alternatives avoid these untoward side effects.

Kava Kava *(Piper methysticum)*

A drink derived from the root of this Polynesian herb (known simply as kava for short) has been used for centuries to reduce anxiety and relax tense muscles. The active components of kava-kava, called *kavalactones,* are concentrated in the root. When compared head-to-head with a benzodiazepine, kava compared favorably to the prescription drug.[12]

Kava is available as a standardized liquid extract or a solid extract in capsules (standardized for kavalactones). Depending on the preparation, take an amount that yields 45 to 70 milligrams of kavalactones, three times daily.

When taken as directed, kava is safe; however, it is contraindicated in patients with depression, pregnant women, and nursing mothers. Kava may also enhance the effect of alcohol and the effectiveness of prescription antidepressant, anti-anxiety, and sedative medications.

Petasites *(Petasites officinalis)*

According to a noted herbalist, petasites is one of the most effective antispasmodic herbs available.[13] This herb relaxes smooth muscle spasms, particularly bladder spasms. The medicinal portions of the plant are the leaves and roots.

The typical dose of petasites is 4.5 to 7 grams of the root or equivalent preparation. Petasites is also available as a fluid extract; take twenty to thirty drops in water, three times daily.

(Note: Since the roots contain potentially harmful substances called pyrollizidine alkaloids, use only alkaloid-free varieties. Petasites is contraindicated in pregnant women and nursing mothers.)

HERBS THAT REDUCE CONSTIPATION

Since constipation increases the pressure on the prostate, it can exacerbate the symptoms of prostatitis. Prevent constipation by drinking plenty of water, exercising, and eating at least 30 grams of fiber daily. If constipation continues, consider trying a short (one to two weeks) trial of the following herbal therapies:

Aloe *(Aloe barbadensis)*

The healing properties of aloe have been known since biblical times. Among other things, one of the ingredients in aloe, called hydroxyanthracene, promotes normal bowel function by increasing fluid accumulation in the intestines and by stimulating intestinal contractions.

Aloe is available as a powder, liquid extract, or juice. The recommended daily dosage of aloe is 20 to 30 milligrams of hydroxyanthracene derivatives (calculated as anhydrous aloin). The proper dose is the smallest dose that maintains soft stools. Limit usage to two weeks.

Although effective, aloe should not be used chronically. Prolonged use makes the bowels "sluggish" and risks electrolyte imbalance (potassium loss) that may interfere with heart medication. Aloe is contraindicated in cases of abdominal pain or obstruction; it is also contraindicated in pregnant women and in children under the age of twelve.

Cascara Sagrada Bark *(Rhamnus purshiana cortex)*

Harvested from the bark of a tree native to the Pacific coast of the United States, Canada, and Eastern Africa, cascara sagrada has the same properties, dosage recommendations (based on hydroxyanthracene derivatives calculated as cascaroside A) and contraindications as aloe. Both preparations should not be taken simultaneously.

Triphala

Consisting of the fruits of three tropical trees, triphala is a popular Ayurvedic (the traditional healing system of India) compound that corrects chronic constipation. Add 5 to 15 grams to a glass of warm water before bedtime (see package label for the appropriate amount). Triphala is also available as a capsule. Take as directed on the package. Available in most health food stores, triphala is safe when taken as directed.

SUPPLEMENTS

In addition to herbal remedies, the following supplements can reduce the incidence and side effects of prostatitis. (For further information on supplements, refer to Appendix A.)

Zinc

The trace mineral zinc is vital to proper immune function and wound healing. Zinc also helps prevent bacterial prostatitis by killing stray bacteria on contact. In contrast to normal men, men with chronic bacterial prostatitis have a low (or even undetectable) zinc concentration within their prostates. This creates a vicious cycle: Infection depresses prostate zinc levels, and depressed prostate zinc levels promote further infection. Unfortunately, once the zinc level becomes depressed, it remains so, even if the infection is gone. Furthermore, the prostate zinc concentration often remains low, even in men taking zinc supplements in high doses.

Even though zinc levels in the prostate may not be improved by supplemental zinc, the zinc level within seminal fluid can be increased by taking supplemental zinc. Infertility, a common side effect of prostatitis, can be improved by taking supplemental zinc.[14]

Zinc is concentrated in oysters, shellfish, and red meat. Zinc supplements are also available. Purchase either zinc gluconate (less expensive) or zinc picolinate (more expensive but better absorbed). Don't take more than 100 milligrams of zinc daily. Excessive zinc competes with copper absorption and depresses the immune system.

D-mannose

D-mannose, a naturally occurring simple sugar that is closely related to glucose, prevents recurrent urinary tract infections. This may seem contradictory, since *refined* sugar depresses immune function. D-mannose, though, works differently. Similar to cranberry juice, D-mannose prevents bacteria *(Escherichia coli)* from adhering to the inner lining of the bladder. If bacteria can't adhere, they can't cause an infection. Although cranberries also contain D-mannose, the amount of D-mannose contained within eight ounces of cranberry juice is only a fraction of the amount contained in half a teaspoon of D-mannose powder.[15]

For patients with recurrent *Escherichia coli* urinary tract infections or prostatitis, I recommend taking half a teaspoon (approximately 2.5 grams) of D-mannose twice daily in a glass of water for prevention, and four times a day during an infection. D-mannose can be taken in addition to prescription antibiotics. Even when taken long-term, D-mannose is safe when taken as directed. (D-mannose is available through Bio Tech Pharmacal, (800) 345-1199.)

Quercetin

Quercetin, a naturally occurring plant flavonoid, significantly decreases prostatitis symptoms by decreasing prostatic inflammation. Flavonoids are plant pigments that give fruits and vegetables their bright colors. In addition to its anti-inflammatory properties, quercetin also inhibits cancer and fights bacterial and fungal infections.

Researchers tested thirty men who randomly received either 500 milligrams of Prosta-Q (a proprietary blend of quercetin and two digestive enzymes called bromelain and papain) twice daily or a placebo for one month.[16] Although few men became totally asymptomatic, two-thirds of the men that were treated with Prosta-Q experienced at least a 25 percent improvement in their prostatitis symptoms versus a 20 percent improvement in the placebo group. Furthermore, inflammatory cells (white blood cells) in the prostatic secretions were improved a mean 68 percent in the Prosta-Q group versus 42 percent in the placebo group. Finally, quercetin decreased oxidative stress within the prostate.

Quercetin is naturally available in foods. Onions, parsley, sage, tomatoes, and citrus fruits are rich sources of quercetin. Although quercetin is also available as a supplement, naturally occurring quercetin is better absorbed than supplemental forms. One way to improve the absorption of supplemental quercetin is to take supplemental bromelain (see page 92) at the same time. The recommended dosage for quercetin is 200 to 400 milligrams twenty minutes before meals three times daily, with an equivalent amount of bromelain. Quercetin is safe when taken as directed.

PROBIOTICS

Probiotics (which means "for life") are "friendly" bacteria and yeast. Most of the more than 400 bacteria that populate the intestinal tract are friendly.

Probiotic Bacteria

Strange as it may sound, friendly intestinal bacteria prevent recurrent infections by neutralizing toxins, crowding out "unfriendly bacteria" (including bacteria that cause recurrent prostatitis such as *E. coli, Proteus vulgaris, Pseudomonas aeruginosa*, and *Streptococcus fecalis*), supporting the immune system, and reducing inflammation.[17] Certain strains of friendly bacteria *(Lactobacilli* and *Bifidobacteria)* also inhibit cancer (including bladder cancer) by inhibiting the growth or activity of cancer-promoting bacteria and by producing chemicals that inhibit cancer growth.[18]

Unfortunately, antibiotics can wipe out friendly intestinal bacteria. As a result, unfriendly bacteria can take over and induce a variety of gastrointestinal problems, including bloating, stomach pain, and diarrhea. Although physicians are familiar with these antibiotic-induced GI side effects, few realize that taking friendly probiotics (such as *Lactobacillus acidophilus,* the kind found in yogurt; *Lactobacillus casei;* and *Bifidobacterium longum*) during and after a course of antibiotic therapy can prevent bothersome intestinal problems.

Give your intestinal tract a good dose of "culture" by eating probiotic-containing foods such as yogurt and sauerkraut (try making your own) and taking supplements that contain friendly probiotic bacteria. Purchase a quality product that has been tested by an independent lab and guaranteed to contain between one and four billion "live, active" organisms per capsule. Also, avoid buying out-of-date products by checking the expiration date on the bottle.

Heat, moisture, and sunlight kill probiotic bacteria. Since the process of compressing probiotics into a tablet generates heat, I recommend choosing a product that has been freeze dried. Available in powder or capsules, probiotics should be stored in the refrigerator in moisture-proof containers. Even if a probiotic is stable at room temperature (many aren't), it should be refrigerated once the container has been opened.

Take probiotics twice daily with food to buffer stomach acid or take an enteric coated brand. The average daily dosage should be between one and ten billion organisms (higher doses can cause stomach upset). Start taking a probiotic the moment you begin taking an antibiotic (but not at the same time), and continue taking it for several weeks after completing the antibiotic.

Probiotic Yeast

In addition to wiping out friendly bacteria, antibiotics can cause an overgrowth of intestinal yeast, which can produce the same unwanted GI side effects as unfriendly bacteria. A special type of yeast, called *Saccharomyces boulardii,* is a certified "yeast-buster." Scientific research has shown that *Saccharomyces boulardii* combats intestinal yeast overgrowth and prevents antibiotic-related intestinal problems by improving intestinal immune function and inactivating bacterial toxins.[19] Purchase a supplement that contains three billion live organisms, and take one capsule twice daily on an empty stomach.

PREBIOTICS

While it may sound like double talk, *prebiotics* are different than *probiotics*. *Prebiotics* are nutrients that supply the friendly bacteria with "health food."

Fructooligosaccharides

Vegetable fiber and complex sugars that are found in certain vegetables promote the growth of friendly bacteria at the expense of unfriendly bacteria. These complex sugars are called fructooligosaccharides (FOS). Foods that contain FOS include soybeans, Jerusalem artichoke, onions, bananas, asparagus, and garlic. A synthetic form of FOS is also available in most health food stores. Since prebiotics support the growth of friendly probiotic bacteria, I recommend taking both supplements together.

The recommended daily dose of FOS ranges between 2,000 and 3,000 milligrams. I encourage patients to eat a generous portion of the foods that are rich in FOS. In addition, since the dietary intake of FOS averages only 800 milligrams daily, I advise patients to supplement their diets with additional FOS to make up the difference.

FOS is available as tablets or as a powder in bulk form or capsules. Powdered FOS that is derived from Jerusalem artichoke has a pleasant nutty flavor. Try sprinkling one to two teaspoons over cereal, salads, or vegetables twice daily.

L-glutamine

The amino acid L-glutamine is another prebiotic that supports normal digestive function. Whenever patients take antibiotics, I recommend taking three grams of L-glutamine daily in divided doses between meals (in addition to taking a probiotic and fructooligosaccharide).

L-glutamine is available in an economical powder (one teaspoon equals three grams) or a more convenient capsule formulation (one capsule typically contains 500 milligrams). L-glutamine can prevent or reverse another antibiotic-related problem called *leaky gut syndrome.*

Leaky gut, or *abnormal intestinal permeability,* occurs whenever the intestinal mucosa (lining) "leaks." Scientists theorize that, left untreated, a leaky gut can cause a variety of health problems, including autoimmune diseases such as arthritis and prostatitis.

VITAMINS

Vitamins are essential to life. Without vitamins, the body's metabolic processes (chemical reactions, food digestion, and detoxification of toxins) would become seriously impaired. Furthermore, without vitamins, our bodies would "rust away" from the harmful effects of oxidation and free radicals. Vitamins are also essential because our bodies can't manufacture them. Therefore, we must obtain vitamins either from the food we eat or by supplementing our diet with vitamin pills.

So how does this relate to prostatitis? Vitamins offset the harmful effects of infection and inflammation, thereby counterbalancing the harmful effects of prostatitis. Infection and inflammation increase oxidant damage within the prostate and generate toxic by-products such as hydroxyl radicals made from hydrogen peroxide. If left unchecked, hydroxyl radicals within the prostate induce inflammation and cause DNA damage.

The prostate defends itself by enlisting the help of an intracellular antioxidant called *glutathione peroxidase* and a related enzyme called *glutathione transferase*. Manufactured by cells throughout the body, glutathione peroxidase renders hydrogen peroxide harmless by converting it to water. This chemical conversion is facilitated by glutathione transferase. In order to do its job, though, glutathione transferase needs the help of vitamin E and the trace mineral selenium. Without these critical cofactors, glutathione transferase fizzles out. When glutathione peroxidase is unable to detoxify hydrogen peroxide to water, hydrogen peroxide is converted into toxic hydroxyl radicals. This creates a dangerous—even life-threatening—situation. In addition to causing prostatitis, hydroxyl radical–induced DNA damage dramatically increases the risk of developing prostate cancer. Supplementing your diet with additional vitamin E and selenium improves glutathione transferase efficiency and significantly reduces the risk of prostate cancer (see pages 135 and 141).

Unfortunately, contrary to popular belief, you can't obtain all the vitamins and minerals that are necessary to achieve optimal health from your diet. The reason is simple: Most diets aren't balanced. They're full of processed foods that are high in fat, salt, and sugar. In fact, Americans derive one-third of their daily calories from junk food. Furthermore, most Americans don't eat the recommended five daily servings of fruits and vegetables.

Therefore, I tell all of my patients, and particularly those with increased demands on their bodies (such as prostatitis), to supplement their diet with a high-potency multivitamin.

HOW OTHER HEALING TRADITIONS TREAT PROSTATITIS

Other holistic healing traditions such as naturopathy, Ayurvedic medicine, homeopathy, and traditional Chinese medicine approach prostatitis differently than do so-called conventional (Western) medicine. In contrast to conventional physicians (who view prostatitis as solely a prostate-related problem), holistic practitioners view prostatitis as an imbalance in the body as a whole.

Holistic healers treat prostatitis by restoring balance within the body. To do this, they cocreate a tailor-made treatment plan with their patients. This treatment plan usually includes many of the natural therapies that I've discussed above. In addition, depending on their specialty, they often employ other therapies, such as acupuncture, specialized dietary instruction, and homeopathic remedies, to name but a few. Unfortunately, space doesn't allow for a detailed discussion of these other healing traditions.

Although the success of other alternative therapies is usually anecdotal (based on personal experience), these therapies have much to offer and deserve further study. I routinely share the care of my difficult prostatitis patients with my alternative medicine colleagues. I've been impressed with the feedback that I've received from these patients.

The Chronic Prostatitis Symptom Index

Use this chart to monitor your progress in the following manner: (1) Calculate and record a separate score for each category (pain, urination, impact of symptoms, and quality of life). (2) Next, calculate and record a "symptom scale score" by adding the pain and urinary scores together (range 0 to 31). Mild = 0 to 9; moderate = 10 to 18; severe = 19 to 31. (3) Finally, calculate a "total score" (range 0 to 43) by totaling the three scores.

NATIONAL INSTITUTES OF HEALTH CHRONIC PROSTATITIS SYMPTOM INDEX

Pain or Discomfort

1. I the last week, have you experienced any pain or discomfort in the following areas:

	Yes	No
a. Areas between rectum and testicles (perineum)	1	0
b. Testicles	1	0
c. Tip of the penis (not related to urination)	1	0
d. Below your waist (in your pubic or bladder area)	1	0

2. In the last week, have you experienced:

	Yes	No
a. Pain or burning during urination	1	0
b. Pain or discomfort during or after ejaculation	1	0

3. How often have you had pain or discomfort in any of these areas over the last week?
- 0 Never
- 1 Rarely
- 2 Sometimes
- 3 Often
- 4 Usually
- 5 Always

4. Which number best describes your AVERAGE pain or discomfort on the days that you have had it over the last week?

0   1   2   3   4   5
(No Pain)

6   7   8   9   10 (Extreme Pain)

Urination

5. How often have you had a sensation of not emptying your bladder completely after you finished urinating, over the last week?
- 0 Not at all
- 1 Less than 1 time in 5
- 2 Less than half the time
- 3 About half the time
- 4 More than half the time
- 5 Almost always

6. How often have you had to urinate less than two hours after you finished urinating, over the last week?
- 0 Not at all
- 1 Less than 1 time in 5
- 2 Less than half the time
- 3 About half the time
- 4 More than half the time
- 5 Almost always

Impact of Symptoms

7. How much have your symptoms kept you from doing the kinds of things you would usually do, over the last week?
- 0 None
- 1 Only a little
- 2 Some
- 3 A lot

8. How much did you think about your symptoms, over the last week?
- 0 None
- 1 Only a little
- 2 Some
- 3 A lot

Quality of Life

9. If you were to spend the rest of your life with your symptoms just the way they have been during the last week, how would you feel about it?
- 0 Delighted
- 1 Pleased
- 2 Mostly satisfied
- 3 Mixed (about equally satisfied and dissatisfied)
- 4 Mostly dissatisfied
- 5 unhappy
- 6 Terrible

Scoring the NIH-Chronic Prostatitis Symptom Index Domains

Pain: Total of items 1a, 1b, 1c, 1d, 2a, 2b, 3 and 4 _____

Urinary Symptoms: Total of items 5 and 6   _____

Quality of Life Impact: Total of items 7, 8 and 9   _____

Reprinted with permission.
Mark W. Litwin et al., "The National Institutes of Health Chronic Prostatitis Symptom Index: Development And Validation of a New Outcome Measure," *Journal of Urology* 162 (August 1999): 374.

How to Measure Your Progress

It's often difficult to determine if you're making any progress. How can you tell if a particular treatment is improving your prostatitis? To address this issue, the National Institutes of Health formulated a simple questionnaire entitled the Chronic Prostatitis Symptoms Index (see page 102).[20]

I encourage my patients to fill out the questionnaire at the end of each week (without referring to their previous answers). You should compare the answers you gave before beginning therapy with your current answers at the end of each month or before changing therapy. The absolute number isn't as important as the trend. If you're not making any progress, discuss the results with your doctor. (Remember, though, that natural therapies work more slowly than prescription drugs. Natural therapies often take six to eight weeks to achieve maximum effectiveness.)

Conclusion

Prostatitis is a poorly understood syndrome that affects millions of American men. Defined mainly by its symptoms, prostatitis affects men of all ages. Unfortunately, conventional treatment for prostatitis, consisting of drugs and surgery, is usually unsuccessful and unrewarding. In contrast, natural remedies for prostatitis can alleviate many of the symptoms of prostatitis—even when conventional therapies have failed. In addition, natural remedies are less expensive, less invasive, and less likely to cause side effects.

Even though natural remedies don't require a doctor's prescription, they shouldn't be considered as a substitute for conventional therapies. Natural remedies and conventional therapies are complementary—they work best when used together. Furthermore, before embarking on a trial of natural therapies for prostatitis, men should undergo a thorough medical evaluation since other conditions can mimic prostatitis.

4

Prostate Cancer

In recent years, the incidence of prostate cancer (abbreviated CaP) has reached epidemic proportions. Although improved methods of diagnosis are cited as one reason for the increase in prostate cancer, there are other factors involved as well. These factors include harmful eating habits, destructive lifestyle choices, and environmental toxins. In this chapter, you'll learn how to modify these risk factors.

First, we'll discuss various aspects of prostate cancer—its incidence, associated risk factors, diagnosis, and conventional treatment. Then we'll look at how natural remedies and conventional therapies for prostate cancer work together.

Types of Prostate Cancer

Prostate cancer is the leading cause of cancer in men—approximately every three minutes, another male in this country is diagnosed with prostate cancer. Currently, over 198,000 men are diagnosed with prostate cancer every year. It comes in two varieties—*clinical* and *latent.*

CLINICAL PROSTATE CANCER

The term *clinical* pertains to the symptoms (complaints like trouble urinating) and to the course of a cancer. Clinical prostate cancer is detected by means of a physical exam, blood test, or X-ray study. If left untreated, clinical prostate cancer can be fatal. Currently, more than 31,000 men die every year because of clinical prostate cancer.

LATENT PROSTATE CANCER

The term *latent* refers to a cancer that is discovered incidentally (when prostate tissue is removed for other reasons). Latent prostate cancer behaves differently from clinical prostate cancer. It's more common, less dangerous, and can't be detected by a physical exam or routine testing. (The incidence of latent prostate cancer is based on autopsy studies.)

As unbelievable as it may seem, researchers have discovered that a small percentage of men start developing latent prostate cancer soon after puberty. Thereafter, the incidence continues to increase with age, so that by age thirty, 30 percent of men have latent cancer cells in their prostates; the figure soars to 60 percent by age forty; and by age eighty, the figure reaches almost 100 percent.[1] Based on these findings, it's estimated that millions of men in this country have latent prostate cancer. Scary as this sounds, the risk of dying from this type of prostate cancer is low.

According to investigators at Johns Hopkins University, a male baby born today has only a 3 percent chance of dying of prostate cancer. The real danger comes when latent prostate cancer cells "wake up" and change into clinical prostate cancer cells—a process that can take as long as thirty years. Although no one knows exactly how, when, or why this happens, new insights into this change have begun to emerge. For instance, research has shown that diet and lifestyle—two items we *can* control—can trigger (or prevent) this lethal scenario.

How Cancer Develops

How cancer develops varies from one individual to another. As a rule, multiple factors are usually involved. Cancer is not just one disease—it's a family of more than 150 different diseases. Prostate cancer arises from cells that line the ducts of the prostate gland. Although 10 percent of prostate cancer is inherited, it usually results from a complex interaction of influences. Our genetic makeup, dietary habits, lifestyle choices, and environmental influences all affect our susceptibility to disease. Regardless of the cause, all cancers develop in three stages—*initiation, promotion,* and *progression.*

INITIATION

Damage to chromosomes, our genetic blueprint, can *initiate* cancer. Fortunately, our bodies are usually able to either repair this damage or program the cancer cells to commit suicide (a process known as *apoptosis*). That's good news, since it's been estimated that each of our body's sixty trillion cells sustains between one thousand and ten thousand DNA "hits" a day. Even so, this cellular repair process isn't perfect—some damaged cells escape and continue to grow. These damaged cells perpetuate the problem by passing faulty information on to the next generation of cells. Ultimately, if this scenario continues, it can lead to cancer.

Carcinogens

Carcinogens are substances that either initiate or promote cancer. Carcinogens increase the risk of cancer by altering communication between cells and interfering with normal cell growth.

Oncogenes are carcinogens that initiate cancer; hence, they're called initiators. Fifty in number, oncogenes ("onco" means cancer; "genes" are a part of the chromosome) initiate cancer by disabling the "brakes" on cell growth.

Tumor suppressor genes reapply the brakes to runaway oncogenes.

Forty in number, suppressor genes slow cell growth by interfering with the cell's growth cycle. Unfortunately, mutations caused by DNA damage can inactivate key tumor suppressor genes. When this happens, without a "governor" to slow them down, cells push the accelerator to the floor and grow like crazy. Mutations in critical suppressor genes can cause cancer. In fact, mutations in a pivotal suppressor gene called "p53" are present in 50 percent of all cancers and in up to 80 percent of prostate cancers.

The other class of carcinogens, called promoters, behaves different from oncogenes. Whereas oncogenes disable the genes that control cell growth, promoters drive cell growth by providing cells with extra fuel. Saturated fat and male hormone (testosterone) are two common promoters that provide prostate cancer cells with high-octane fuel.

PROMOTION

The next intersection on the road to cancer is called the *promotion* stage. Unlike the initiation stage (which is reversible), the promotion stage is permanent. Once the mutation becomes incorporated into precursor cells (called "stem cells"), there's no turning back.

Cancer cells grow by doubling. Like a cookie cutter, cancer cells make copies of themselves. This process of cancer growth is called "doubling." The time it takes a tumor to double in size, called the doubling time, varies from one tumor to another. The faster the doubling time, the faster the tumor growth. Although prostate cancer cells can double as quickly as every two weeks, or as slowly as every ten years, most prostate cancer cells cruise at speeds somewhere in between. The concept of doubling time will become important when we discuss therapies for prostate cancer.

Unfortunately, tumors are too small to be seen or felt at the time when treatment is most effective—early in the promotion process. Until a tumor has grown to the size of a dime, it's invisible to most of the modern diagnostic equipment. In fact, even the most advanced equipment won't detect a tumor until it has doubled thirty times and reached a population of a billion cells or more!

Fortunately, prostate tumors are not like other tumors. In the case of prostate cancer, a simple blood test, called prostatic specific antigen (PSA), can detect tumor cells years before they're detectable by other means. Like radar, PSA detects speeding tumor cells long before they're seen.

PROGRESSION

This last part of the journey is the most perilous and often results in the death of the host. Up to this point, cancer cells, like normal cells, have stayed on the main highway. Normal cells stay put, grow at a predictable rate, and die once their work is done. Cancer cells play by different rules—they're immortal, can *progress* or invade surrounding tissue, and spread to other parts of the body (metastasize).

As you'll soon learn, natural remedies sidetrack cancer cells by preventing or reversing the stage of initiation and putting the brakes on the stages of tumor promotion and progression.

Risk Factors

While nobody knows exactly what causes prostate cancer, researchers have determined that a complex interplay of different risk factors increases the chance of developing prostate cancer. These are discussed below. Fortunately, as you'll learn later in this chapter, you can modify these risk factors by making key lifestyle and dietary modifications.

FAMILY HISTORY

Perhaps the most important risk factor for prostate cancer is a family history. In the United States, approximately a quarter of the cases of prostate cancer are due to genetic clustering—that is, more than one family member has a history of prostate cancer (19 percent of these men have *hereditary* prostate cancer versus 81 percent with *familial* prostate cancer).

Familial Prostate Cancer

Familial prostate cancer is simply a clustering of prostate cancer within families. In either case, the odds of developing prostate cancer escalate as the number of family members with prostate cancer increases. For instance, in the case of familial prostate cancer, if one first-degree relative has prostate cancer, the risk is two to three times greater; with two first-degree relatives, it's five to six times greater; and with three, it's eight to eleven times greater. If a second-degree relative (uncle or grandfather on either side of the family) has prostate cancer, there's still a one and a half to two times greater risk. If two second-degree relatives have prostate cancer, the risk is nine times greater.

Hereditary Prostate Cancer

Hereditary prostate cancer is suspected when there is a history of prostate cancer affecting family members within three generations, three first-degree relatives (brothers and father), or two relatives before the age of fifty-five.

Men who inherit a dominant gene for prostate cancer have a sixteen to eighteen times greater chance of developing prostate cancer. This equates to an 80 to 90 percent chance of developing prostate cancer by age eighty-five. The gene is also passed from father to daughter. This means that a son can inherit the prostate cancer gene from his mother. Although the gene has been identified, at this point there isn't a blood test to screen for genetic prostate cancer.

Family History of Breast Cancer

Men have a threefold greater risk of developing prostate cancer if they carry the breast cancer gene *(BRCA1)*. The risk of prostate cancer is also increased in men whose sisters have breast cancer.

POOR LIFESTYLE HABITS

Poor lifestyle habits, as discussed throughout this book, can also increase the risk of prostate cancer. These include high-fat diet, obesity, smoking, excessive alcohol consumption, and lack of exercise.

ELEVATED LEVELS OF
INSULIN-LIKE GROWTH FACTOR-1

Originating in the liver, insulin-like growth factor-1 (abbreviated IGF-1) causes cells to grow and prevents *apoptosis* (programmed cell death). According to one study, men with the highest levels of IGF-1 had a four and a half times greater risk of developing prostate cancer; for those over the age of sixty, the risk was *eightfold*.[2] IGF-1 also stimulates prostate cancer cells to make a substance that promotes tumor cell growth (called urokinase-type plasminogen activator). Finally, IGF-1 increases tumor growth by supporting angiogenesis (the formation of new blood vessels).

OCCUPATION

Your workplace can be hazardous in more ways than one. Certain occupations increase the risk of developing prostate cancer. For instance, farmers have a higher incidence of prostate cancer than the general population, as do men who work in the rubber, textile, chemical, drug, fertilizer, and atomic energy industries.

CHEMICALS AND TOXINS

Any chemical or toxin that is foreign to the body is known as a *xenobiotic*. Pesticides and herbicides (weedkillers) are two common examples that heighten the risk of prostate cancer by causing DNA damage and altering hormone metabolism. In the year 2000, the Environmental Protection Agency upgraded *atrazine*—the most commonly used herbicide in the United States—from a "possible" to a "probable" cause of cancer (including prostate cancer).[3] Atrazine is used on corn, sorghum, and citrus crops. In addition, Vietnam veterans who were exposed to the now-banned Agent Orange (dioxin) have an increased risk of developing prostate cancer.

Endocrine disrupters—substances that mimic natural hormones—also increase the risk of prostate cancer. Common examples of endocrine disrupters include polychlorinated biphenols, or PCBs (used to make plastic, ink, as well as electrical and electronic equipment), and plasticizers (substances used to make plastic food-wrap more pliable).

Finally, in addition to being high in fat, dairy and beef products are often contaminated with toxic pesticide and hormone residues. (That's why the European Common Market bans the importation of U.S. dairy and beef products.)

GEOGRAPHY

Studies have shown that sunlight (just fifteen minutes per day) can prevent prostate cancer by stimulating the body to make vitamin D. Researchers have discovered that vitamin D prevents prostate cancer cells from growing.

Certain mineral deficiencies also increase the odds of developing prostate cancer. For example, men who live in regions of the country where the soil is deficient in the trace mineral selenium have a higher incidence and death rate from prostate cancer.

RACE AND NATIONALITY

Unfortunately, African-American males in this country have the highest incidence of prostate cancer in the world. Although many theories have been proposed, the reason remains unclear. While one's race can't be changed, unhealthy lifestyle and dietary choices can be.

Like race, the incidence of prostate cancer varies greatly from one country to another. China has the lowest incidence, Switzerland the highest, with the United States falling somewhere in between. Researchers attribute these international differences more to diet than genetics. For instance, a typical Chinese diet is rich in cancer-preventing foods such as soy protein and low in cancer-promoting foods such as animal fat. A typical Swiss diet is the reverse.

VASECTOMY

According to some researchers, men who've had a vasectomy have an increased risk of developing prostate cancer. In contrast, after carefully reviewing the data from fourteen observational studies between 1988 and 1996, other researchers concluded that there is *not* an association between vasectomy and prostate cancer.[4] Similarly, the American Urologic Association and the National Institutes of Health have reached the same conclusion that vasectomy and prostate cancer risk is unrelated.

Diagnosis of Prostate Cancer

While examining a tissue sample under the microscope is the only sure way to make the diagnosis of prostate cancer, information obtained from a patient's history, physical exam, blood tests, and X-ray studies often suggests its presence.

SIGNS AND SYMPTOMS OF PROSTATE CANCER

Although often asymptomatic, men with prostate cancer may experience a variety of signs and symptoms. *Signs* are physical findings, like blood in the semen. *Symptoms* are complaints, like difficulty urinating. Signs and symptoms are often indicative of an underlying disease and warrant further investigation. The signs and symptoms of prostate cancer can be divided into three main categories: problems related to *bladder outflow obstruction* (difficulty urinating), *local tumor involvement,* and *metastatic disease.*

Bladder Outflow Obstruction

Men with prostate cancer often come to their physician complaining of a change in their voiding or urinary habits. For instance, they may complain of a poor urine flow, trouble starting their stream, frequent and urgent urination, and a sensation of incomplete emptying of their bladder. Although prostate cancer can cause these symptoms, it is not the most common cause—prostate infection or enlargement is usually to blame. Just the same, a change in voiding habits should prompt a visit to the doctor.

Local Tumor Involvement

As prostate cancer grows, it may irritate or even invade the urethra. When this happens, men often experience blood in the urine, burning on urination, or obstruction of the urine flow (urinary retention). If the tumor extends outside the prostate, it can damage the nerves that surround the prostate, causing impotence. The tumor can also extend into or beneath the bladder and squeeze shut the ureters or invade the seminal vesicles (causing blood to appear in the semen).

Metastatic Disease

Once prostate cancer escapes the prostate, it can travel to other areas in the body. One of its favorite landing sites is the bone marrow (the site where new blood cells are formed). In its new location, prostate cancer wreaks havoc by destroying bone marrow cells and weakening the overlying bone. Consequently, metastatic prostate cancer often causes anemia (low blood count), bone fractures (breaks), and bone pain (due to local tumor growth).

Although it's important to see your physician if you have any of the above signs and symptoms, it's best to detect prostate cancer before they appear. Fortunately, millions of men are getting the message. Thanks to the effective use of three diagnostic tests—the *prostate specific antigen (PSA) blood test, digital rectal exam* (abbreviated DRE), and *transrectal prostate ultrasound* (abbreviated TRUS)—the chance of detecting cancer before it has spread is now better than ever before.

PSA BLOOD TEST

PSA screening consists of three components: a simple questionnaire about the presence or absence of signs and symptoms of prostate cancer, a DRE, and a PSA blood test. PSA screening detects 70 percent of new cases of prostate cancer when they're still confined to the prostate, as compared to 35 percent of the cases in the pre-PSA era. Cancers that are detected early enough when they are still confined to the prostate have a much better chance of being cured. Studies have also shown that the majority (93 percent) of prostate cancers that are detected as a result of PSA screening are significant; that is, if left untreated, they'll progress.

PSA screening should be done yearly starting at age forty for men with suspected hereditary prostate, at age forty-five for men in the high-risk group, and at age fifty for all other men. Routine PSA screening, though, is not recommended for men over the age of seventy-five or for those with a life expectancy of less than ten years.

The PSA is interpreted in several ways. First is the "Total PSA." Detected by a simple blood test, a Total PSA (usually referred to simply as a "PSA" value or level) measures the total amount of PSA in the bloodstream. Approximately 90 percent of the PSA in the blood is bound or stuck to another protein; the remaining portion is unbound. An elevated PSA is an early warning sign of cancer. A normal PSA value is 4 nanograms per milliliter (abbreviated ng/ml) or less (range of zero to four); an elevated PSA level is greater than 4 ng/ml. Just the same, an elevated PSA doesn't necessarily mean that a patient has prostate cancer. Only one-third of men with an elevated PSA are diagnosed with prostate cancer.

Furthermore, PSA can be elevated for reasons other than cancer. For instance, an enlarged prostate, prostate infection (prostatitis), or having sex within twenty-four hours of the blood test can elevate the PSA level. In addition, duplicate PSA values can vary by as much as 20 percent— even when using automated equipment from the same laboratory. Finally, PSA values increase with age.

In an effort to improve the accuracy of PSA testing, researchers have experimented with other applications of PSA. One modification is called *age-adjusted PSA*. Younger men have lower PSA values than older men; however, the same normal reference range (0 to 4 ng/ml) is used for both age groups. Consequently, prostate cancer may be missed in younger men, while unnecessary prostate biopsies may be performed in older men. In order to rectify this situation, some researchers recommend using an age-specific PSA reference range. Normal age-specific PSA values are as follows:[5]

- Men aged 40 to 49: 2.5 ng/ml or less
- Men aged 50 to 59: 3.5 ng/ml or less
- Men aged 60 to 69: 4.5 ng/ml or less
- Men aged 70 to 79: 6.5 ng/ml or less

Researchers have also discovered that normal PSA levels vary among Caucasian and African-American men. According to one study, the adjusted "Caucasian-based" ranges listed above would have missed 40 percent of African-American men with prostate cancer! Accordingly, the study recommends an age-specific reference range for African-American men as follows:[6]

- Men aged 40 to 49: 2 ng/ml or less
- Men aged 50 to 59: 4 ng/ml or less
- Men aged 60 to 69: 4.5 ng/ml or less
- Men aged 70 to 79: 5.5 ng/ml or less

Finally, there is another measure of the PSA, called the "percentage-free PSA." This modification of PSA measures the ratio between total PSA (bound and unbound) and the unbound, or "free," PSA in the serum. This test is most useful for men with PSA levels between 4 and 10. According to some reports, the percentage-free PSA is more accurate than PSA alone in predicting the presence of prostate cancer. As the percentage-free PSA decreases, the chance of cancer increases. For instance, a man aged fifty to sixty-four, with a PSA between 4 and 10 ng/ml and a percentage-free PSA of greater than 25 percent, has a less than 5 percent chance of harboring prostate cancer. If his percentage-free fraction is 10 percent or less, the chance of finding prostate cancer jumps to 56 percent.

There is one drawback to using percentage-free PSA, though: All forms of prostate manipulation, even a rectal examination, alter the percentage-free fraction. Therefore, a percentage-free PSA blood test should not be drawn on the same day following a rectal examination or within twenty-four hours of sexual intercourse.

DIGITAL RECTAL EXAM

A simple office procedure that takes only seconds to perform, a DRE is performed by inserting a lubricated gloved finger inside the rectum (see Figure 2.2 on page 33). This allows your doctor to feel the outside surface of the prostate (called the peripheral zone). Since approximately 70 percent of prostate cancers arise from the peripheral zone, an abnormal DRE is often the first sign of prostate cancer.

Men often ask if they can skip the DRE and just get a PSA blood test. The answer is an emphatic NO! PSA screening, while useful, should not be used alone. Studies have shown that up to one-third of men with prostate cancer—particularly the most aggressive type—*have normal PSA values.*

If an abnormality is found on DRE, or if the PSA level is elevated, your primary physician will refer you to a urologist—a specialist who can diagnose and treat prostate cancer. The next step is usually a TRUS.

TRANSRECTAL PROSTATE ULTRASOUND (TRUS)

In this test, a special ultrasound probe that emits sound waves is inserted into the rectum. These reflected sound waves are then displayed on a TV monitor that allows your urologist to see the internal portions of the prostate. If an abnormality is detected, a biopsy (sample) of the suspicious area is taken by inserting a needle through a separate channel located within the probe. Prostate tissue obtained by a TRUS-guided biopsy is sent to a laboratory for further evaluation. A specialist, called a pathologist, examines the tissue under a microscope. If cancer cells are detected (a "positive" biopsy), the pathologist's report will include information about the tumor size (estimated by the number and extent of biopsy specimens that contains tumor) and aggressiveness (based on the Gleason score, see below).

INTERPRETING BIOPSY TEST RESULTS

Tumor cells are graded by their appearance under the microscope and are rated according to the *Gleason score,* which has a range from 2 to 10. The higher the score, the more aggressive the tumor. Aggressive tumors—those with a Gleason score of 7 or above—are more likely to spread.

Before your doctor can make a recommendation regarding treatment, other factors must be considered. These include the PSA level (the higher the PSA reading, the greater the risk for spread) and the tumor stage (extent of the cancer).

Accurate tumor staging prevents the inappropriate use of invasive therapies when there is little chance for cure—that is, when the tumor has already spread to other parts of the body. There are two types of staging—*clinical* staging (based on the results of the prostate biopsy, DRE, plus other blood and X-ray tests) and *pathologic* staging (based on an examination of surgically removed tissue).

Clinical Staging

Clinical staging uses a system called *TNM,* which stands for tumor (T), lymph nodes (N), and metastasis (M). The primary tumor stage is subdivided into four stages, designated T1 through T4. Cancers that are confined to the prostate are labeled as T1–T2. Tumors that have spread outside the prostate, or into structures that surround the prostate, are designated as T3–T4.

If the tumor has spread to the lymph nodes, it's designated as N+; if it has metastasized further, it's designated as M+. When there's a high likelihood that the tumor has spread beyond the prostate (for instance, when men have a prostate cancer with a Gleason score of 7 or higher or a PSA level that is greater than 20), additional staging studies are usually ordered.

Pathologic Staging

In addition to examining tissue under the microscope, the pathologic stage can be estimated by using special tables called nomograms. The best known of these tables, called the Partin nomogram, was devised by comparing the pathologic stage of thousands of surgical specimens with the preoperative clinical stage (DRE, Gleason score, and PSA). The Partin nomogram is available on the Internet courtesy of the Prostate Cancer Research Institute: http://www.prostate-cancer.org.

If the biopsy report comes back showing cancer, your doctor will sit down with you and discuss the risks and benefits associated with each of the various options used to treat prostate cancer. During this office visit, you will be bombarded with an incredible amount of information. To help cope with this information overload, I suggest you take someone along— a loved one or friend—to take notes. A tape recorder is also handy.

You should also ask questions. If you don't understand something, ask enough questions until you do. Ask for copies of your biopsy and test results. Start making a file. Remember, this is your life being discussed, not some obscure statistic.

Remember that you have plenty of time to sift through the information your doctor has just presented. (Prostate cancer is generally a slow-growing tumor.) If you still have questions, make another appointment with your physician to discuss the matter. Making an informed choice, one based on knowledge of the various options weighed against the risks and benefits, is the most important decision you may ever have to make.

Never forget that *you,* not your doctor, have the final say in any decision. If you feel pressured to make a decision, if the one recommended doesn't agree with you, or if you are still uncertain, consider getting a second opinion. Seeking a second opinion merely allows another physician to review your case and render an independent opinion. This opinion, by the way, may or may not agree with your doctor's recommendation. You'll be relieved to know that seeking a second opinion does not mean that you'll need another prostate biopsy, or even additional testing in most cases.

Conventional Therapies for Prostate Cancer

What is the best treatment for localized prostate cancer? This vexing question haunts every patient who confronts prostate cancer. Urologists also wrestle with the same question. The truth is, there isn't a "best" treatment for prostate cancer. It varies from one individual to another depending on a variety of factors, such as the clinical stage of the cancer, the age and life expectancy, and the tolerance for risking complications such as urinary incontinence and impotence.

After considering these variables, your doctor will recommend one of the following four options: *watchful waiting, surgery, radiation therapy*—either external beam and/or brachytherapy (radioactive seeds)—and *cryotherapy* (freezing the prostate). A brief overview of each of these options is discussed below.

WATCHFUL WAITING

Watchful waiting is also discussed in Chapter 2. Just as the phrase implies, it means that no further treatment—other than careful observation—is planned. While watchful waiting remains controversial, most researchers agree that, under certain circumstances, it is appropriate. Men with a life expectancy of less than ten years due to age or medical problems might benefit from this conservative treatment, as will men over the age of seventy with slow-growing tumors (Gleason of 2 to 4 or slow doubling time). But this course of treatment isn't recommended for everyone. In particular, it is not recommended for healthy men under the age of seventy with tumors confined to the prostate. For one thing, all prostate cancers, if left untreated, will continue to grow, and there is no way to accurately predict at what point it will spread beyond the prostate and become incurable. Also, about one-third of all prostate tumors are *understaged,* meaning they are more extensive or aggressive than shown on the biopsy report.

If you are less than age seventy when you're diagnosed, have a higher PSA, or if there's cancer felt during the rectal exam, then additional treatment is recommended.

PROSTATE SURGERY

Developed around the turn of this century, surgical removal of the prostate, also called *radical prostatectomy,* is currently the most popular treatment for localized prostate cancer.

Two different surgical approaches are used to remove the prostate. One approach, called a *radical retropubic prostatectomy,* is performed through an incision made from the belly button to the pubic bone. Another approach, called a *radical perineal prostatectomy,* is performed through an incision made in the skin between the anus and scrotum. In both cases, the prostate and seminal vesicles are removed. Since prostate cancer can spread to the pelvic lymph nodes, this tissue is usually removed as well. The technique chosen depends on the surgeon's training. Both techniques work equally well.

The surgery is performed on the same day of admission to the hospital and takes about two to three hours. After a three-day hospital stay, a catheter remains in place for another ten days. Return to normal activity is usually possible after three to four weeks of convalescence.

According to a report from Johns Hopkins University, approximately 85 percent of men with stages T1 and T2 tumors, and 43 percent of men with T3 tumors, treated with surgery are free of disease (cured) at ten years.[7]

Surgery offers certain advantages that are not offered by the other therapies used to treat prostate cancer. At least theoretically, surgery removes all the cancer from the body. Unlike nonsurgical therapies for prostate cancer, tissue is examined under the microscope. Men who experience difficult urination before surgery (due to an enlarged prostate) usually experience significant improvement in their voiding symptoms after surgery. And, without a prostate, the PSA should be nondetectable.

However, in spite of its many advantages, radical prostatectomy has its complications, which can occur early after the procedure or later. Early complications include blood loss and infection. Late complications include urinary incontinence and impotence, which increase in older patients. Fortunately, urinary incontinence is usually temporary—over 50 percent of men regain continence by three months following surgery, and all but 5 percent of the remaining men regain control within a year. There are new devices to help cope with both of these complications. (See "Dealing with Incontinence and Impotence" on page 122.)

RADIATION THERAPY

First discovered in 1895, X-rays have been used to treat prostate cancer since 1910. Radiation therapy (abbreviated RT) uses high-energy photons (X rays) or heavy particle beams (neutrons and protons) to either directly or indirectly damage cellular DNA. Tumor cells either stop growing or undergo apoptosis when their DNA is damaged.

Dealing with Incontinence and Impotence

Men with severe urinary incontinence are often miserable. Fortunately, they can become dry again thanks to an innovative medical device called an *artificial genitourinary sphincter*. Used on an outpatient basis, this nifty three-component device consists of a thin collar (about the size of a tape measure) that is surgically placed around the urethra; a small pump (about the size of a big jelly bean) that is placed just beneath the skin in the scrotum; and a reservoir (about the size of a Ping-Pong ball) that is placed in the lower abdomen. Except during urination, fluid in the collar exerts sufficient pressure around the urethra to prevent incontinence. During urination, the fluid in the collar is transferred to the reservoir by pressing a release valve on the pump. After urination, the fluid is recycled into the collar, and continence is restored. This device is usually reserved for men with severe incontinence that persists for at least one year following surgery (since the incontinence may improve on its own).

More men, however, are affected with impotence than urinary incontinence. Even so, when the nerves surrounding the prostate are "spared," approximately 60 percent of men (who were potent beforehand) maintain their potency after surgery. It can take up to a year for men to regain their potency following radical prostate surgery, because the nerves are often bruised during the procedure.

Oral medications (such as Viagra), injectable medications (such as prostaglandin E1), and *vacuum tumescence pumps* (devices that cause penile swelling by creating a vacuum) can correct impotence by increasing penile blood flow. Another device, called a *penile prosthesis,* bypasses the need for additional penile blood flow altogether. Performed as an outpatient surgical procedure, two silicone cylinders are positioned within the penis inside the space that normally expands with blood during an erection. A pump in the scrotum is compressed to transfer fluid from a reservoir to the pair of cylinders in the penis to get an erection; likewise, a release valve is pressed to return the penis to a normal state.

Performed on an outpatient basis, RT is delivered to the prostate by means of an external machine (hence the name "external beam" therapy).

Lasting fifteen to thirty minutes each, a series of five daily treatments are given weekly for six to seven weeks.

The chief advantage of RT is that surgery is not required. Most men can continue with their normal activities throughout therapy. However, RT can also cause complications. For instance, RT can cause urinary complications such as difficulty voiding or burning on urination; bowel problems such as diarrhea or rectal pain; and impotence in 60 percent of men who were potent beforehand.

RT can also significantly increase the risk of secondary malignancies, especially of the bladder.[8] Overall, compared to nonradiated patients, men who receive radiation therapy to the prostate have a 15 percent greater chance of developing bladder cancer. Even though the absolute number of men who develop bladder cancer is only 1 percent or so, the risk of developing bladder cancer increases as a function of time. Fortunately, as you will soon discover, natural therapies can decrease the risk of developing these radiation-induced cancers.

The success of RT is determined by measuring the PSA value. Before starting RT, most patients have an elevated PSA level (greater than 4). Following radiation therapy, the PSA level usually reaches its lowest level within eighteen months, although it can rise again temporarily. According to researchers from Massachusetts General Hospital, the chance for cure after ten years following RT was 91 percent if the PSA was less than .5 nanograms per milliliter (ng/ml); 86 percent if the PSA was between .5 and 1 ng/ml; and 74 percent if the PSA was between 1 and 2 ng/ml.[9] Prostate cancer recurrences following RT are rare after ten years.

BRACHYTHERAPY

Brachytherapy is an outpatient surgical procedure in which tiny radioactive seeds (usually iodine-125 or paladium-103) are implanted into the prostate gland. "Brachy" means short—the radioactive seeds release their radiation over a short distance, as opposed to external beam RT, which affects a much broader area.

Brachytherapy is an outpatient surgical procedure that is performed under general anesthesia. A transrectal ultrasound probe is used to guide the placement of special needles—usually twenty-five or so—into various areas of the prostate. These needles are poked through the skin in the perineum (the area between the anus and the scrotal sac)—a surgical incision isn't necessary.

Approximately 70 to 150 seeds, each about the size of a grain of rice, are implanted throughout the prostate. The seeds give off intense radiation to an area measuring about the size of a dime. Although the seeds are permanent, they release most of their radiation within a year (ranging between three and twelve months, depending on the type of seed that's used).

The entire procedure takes about an hour. Normal activity can usually be resumed within a matter of a few days.

The chief advantage of brachytherapy is that it can be performed as a single outpatient procedure. However, many of the same side effects associated with other therapies are also encountered with brachytherapy. Furthermore, data on long-term cure rates are still preliminary.

Following brachytherapy, approximately two-thirds of men are cured at ten years (PSA less than 0.5 ng/ml).

CRYOTHERAPY

Cryotherapy, also called *cryoablation,* was first used to treat prostate cancer in 1964. Delivered through special probes inserted into the prostate, liquid nitrogen or helium/neon is used to freeze the prostate. Although promising, cryosurgery is still considered experimental by most urologists. Cryosurgery is usually reserved for men with high-stage, high-grade tumors and locally recurrent prostate cancer following RT.

TREATMENTS FOR LOCALLY ADVANCED
PROSTATE CANCER

When the cancer has grown just outside the prostate but nowhere else, it's called locally advanced prostate cancer (Stage T3). Unfortunately, other than surgery—where the tissue around the prostate can be microscopically examined—most tests are unreliable at predicting the presence or absence of cancer cells just outside the prostate gland. As a result, many tumors are understaged. In fact, after surgery, about 50 percent of men felt to have T2 disease (tumor confined to the prostate) are found instead to have T3 disease (tumor outside the prostate).

Although the best management for locally advanced prostate cancer remains controversial, treatment often involves some type of surgery or radiation therapy.

TUMOR RECURRENCE

In some cases, prostate cancer returns even though the original therapy appeared to cure it. The best way to proceed in this situation is hotly debated among cancer specialists. Some favor immediate and aggressive treatment; others recommend conservative management (no treatment). Nobody knows for sure which approach is best.

Before determining which way to proceed, the risks and benefits of therapy must be weighed against a number of factors. These factors include the patient's age, medical condition, time interval between primary therapy and PSA failure, PSA doubling time, "risk factors" for recurrent disease, and, most important, quality-of-life priorities.

In the final analysis, treatment depends on whether the recurrence is localized or metastatic. In the case of locally recurrent prostate cancer, most urologists recommend radiation therapy. Studies have shown that early treatment in this situation offers the best chance for cure.

If the prostate cancer is metastatic, *androgen-deprivation therapy* or chemotherapy is often used (see below). Early treatment reduces the incidence of serious complications, such as bone fractures and paralysis due to spinal cord compression. Furthermore, if the metastatic disease is minimal, early treatment also improves survival.

ANDROGEN-DEPRIVATION THERAPY

Androgen-deprivation therapy—one of the mainstays for treating metastatic prostate cancer—uses drugs or surgery to prevent androgen (a male hormone) from stimulating prostate cancer cells. Androgen is produced in the testicles and in the adrenal glands. Some prostate cancer cells need this male hormone to grow. They commit suicide if they are deprived of it. Approximately 80 percent of prostate cancer cells fall into this category. Prostate cancer cells that have "escaped" the need for male hormone no longer require male hormone to grow. Therefore, depriving androgen-resistant cancer cells of androgen has little effect.

A variety of methods are used to halt male hormone production. These include removing the testicles (called an *orchiectomy*) and taking medication—either a shot (which stops the testicles from making male hormone) or a pill, called an *anti-androgen* (which blocks the effect of androgens at the cellular level).

Although effective and often lifesaving, androgen-deprivation therapy can cause a variety of side effects, including anemia, hot flashes (sudden sweating and flushing), fatigue, mood swings, liver damage, and osteoporosis. As you'll learn in the next section, natural therapies can minimize some of these side effects.

CHEMOTHERAPY

When most people think of chemotherapy (drug therapy used to treat cancer), they envision the horror stories they've heard about or witnessed. Although chemotherapy can have serious side effects, modern chemotherapy is currently one of the most promising areas in prostate cancer research. Surprising as it may seem, these recent advances are not the result of revolutionary new drugs. They're the result of using existing drugs in novel ways.

Combination chemotherapy allows oncologists (medical specialists who treat cancer) to treat prostate cancer more effectively. It works like this: Cytoxic ("cyto" means cell) chemotherapy kills cancer cells by interfering with various phases of their growth cycle. For instance, alkylating agents such as Estramustine (brand name Emcyt) and mitotic inhibitors such as paclitaxel (brand name Taxol) throw a monkey wrench in prostate cancer cell growth by interfering with its DNA replication. When used together, these two drugs are more effective than either agent used alone.

In other words, by combining drugs that work together, oncologists are able to deliver a one-two knockout punch before cancer cells know what hit them. Furthermore, by using drugs that work together, it's often possible to lower the dose of individual medications and decrease the side effects.

Finally, regardless of whether the disease is locally recurrent or metastatic, natural therapies for prostate cancer, which will be discussed in the next section, should be part of every treatment protocol.

CANCER CLINICAL TRIALS

Currently, more than sixty FDA-approved clinical trials are investigating options for treating recurrent prostate cancer. Cancer clinical trials test new cancer treatments in people with cancer. For example, clinical trials test new drugs, new approaches to surgery or radiation, new combinations of therapies, or innovations such as gene therapy. Trials consist of three phases.

As with any treatment, before agreeing to participate in a cancer clinical trial, you should weigh the possible risks against the potential benefits. These benefits may include:

- the opportunity to receive state-of-the art treatment
- a chance to benefit from the latest medical advances
- the possibility of advancing medical research

There are possible risks of participating in a clinical trial. For instance:

- New treatments may not be as effective as standard treatments or may be associated with unexpected side effects.
- Even if the new treatment is beneficial, it may not be effective for an individual patient.
- Patients may be randomized (assigned) to the standard treatment or a placebo treatment (inactive pill or treatment) rather than the new treatment.
- There may be unexpected costs.

Unfortunately, only 3 percent of eligible cancer patients participate in clinical trials. Why? Most people are unaware that these trials exist, or if they are aware, they assume that they aren't eligible to participate. If you want to find out more about clinical trials for prostate cancer, talk to your doctor or contact the NCI (National Cancer Institute) for a comprehensive listing of NCI-sponsored clinical trials (CancerNet@http://cancernet.nci.nih.gov/)

Natural Remedies for Prostate Cancer

While most physicians aren't aware that natural remedies can complement conventional cancer therapies, their patients know better. According to an article that appeared in the journal *Cancer,* one-third of cancer patients (ranging between 7 and 64 percent) use alternative therapies.[10] This trend applies to men with prostate cancer as well.

I strongly believe that *all* men with prostate cancer should use the natural remedies that are discussed below. Why? Perhaps the words of Michael Lerner, author of *Choices in Healing,* sum it up best: "Patients [who use complementary therapies] achieve higher quality of life, respond better to most conventional cancer therapies, experience fewer side effects of treatment and fewer symptoms of disease, control pain better with less need for medication, experience more lasting or partial remissions and, if they die, experience better deaths."[11]

Cancer doesn't occur overnight. It's a dynamic process; it's constantly evolving and potentially reversible. As we learned in the first section, cancer cells originate from normal cells that have been altered because of dietary, lifestyle, genetic, and environmental influences. Cells that have already accumulated one or more cancer risk factors are particularly susceptible to malignant transformation.

Since cancer cells (like normal cells) continually adapt to changes in their local environment, it may be possible to slow down or even reverse cancer by altering these risk factors.

Finally, unhealthy eating habits and lifestyle choices can be a time bomb, *even for men who supposedly have been cured of prostate cancer.* Years later, if any stray cancer cells remain, they can be reactivated by cancer-promoting dietary and lifestyle habits.[12]

In the following pages, I'll discuss how healthy lifestyle and dietary choices, along with selective vitamins, herbs, and nutritional supplements, can slow down or prevent the initiation, promotion, and progression stages of prostate cancer.

LIFESTYLE MODIFICATIONS

Lifestyle—how we live—can either increase or decrease the risk of prostate cancer. (Many of the lifestyle changes listed in Chapters 2 and 3 also apply here. See pages 49 and 50 and pages 72–75, respectively.) Obvious modifications like decreasing stress, getting plenty of aerobic exercise, losing weight, avoiding excessive alcohol and tobacco, and avoiding environmental toxins are all steps that you can take to improve the overall health of your prostate and your body.

DIET

Even though the age-adjusted incidence of *latent* prostate cancer in native Japanese and American males is roughly the same, *clinical* prostate cancer is twentyfold higher in American males. Researchers attribute this glaring discrepancy to dietary differences. A Japanese diet is high in soy protein and fish but low in fat from dairy and red meat. The exact opposite is true of a typical American diet.

As further proof, according to scientific research, once Japanese males adopt a "standard American diet" (euphemistically known as "SAD"), their incidence of *clinical* prostate cancer goes up tenfold. In other words, even though cancer cells are present in both situations, a Japanese-type diet prevents prostate cancer cells from becoming activated. A Japanese-type diet also decreases the risk of dying from prostate cancer.

Establishing healthy eating habits is one of the best ways to prevent prostate cancer. You can immediately start lowering your risk of prostate cancer by adopting the suggestions made in each of the following categories:

Fat

As discussed in Chapters 2 and 3, reducing the amount of fat in your diet, particularly saturated animal fat, is one of the best changes you can make. Among other things, excess fat can triple the risk of prostate cancer. Eliminate or greatly reduce junk snack foods and red meat.

Men who eat red meat have twice the risk of prostate cancer. (See "The Arachidonic Acid Cascade" on page 131 for details.) Dairy products are also high in saturated fat. Many contain traces of recombinant bovine growth hormone, a genetically engineered hormone that is used to increase milk production, which increases the risk of prostate cancer by as much as eightfold by increasing the production of IGF-1 (see page 111). Creamy salad dressings, nuts, and fatty farm-raised fish such as salmon are all high-fat foods that should be limited or avoided altogether.

Oils

Safflower, corn, cottonseed, soybean, peanut oil, flaxseed, and canola oil contain fatty acids that increase arachidonic acid and inflammatory eicosanoid production, which increases the risk of prostate cancer. Use olive oil instead. A diet rich in olive oil decreases the risk of prostate cancer.

Fruits and Vegetables

In addition to all kinds of fruits and vegetables, the following deserve special mention:

- **Tomatoes.** They are rich in *lycopene,* a cancer-fighting antioxidant vitamin that gives them the red color. Harvard researchers found that eating tomatoes at least four times weekly lowers the risk of prostate cancer by 20 percent, and eating ten weekly helpings lowers the risk by 45 percent.[13] (A serving is one-half cup of raw or cooked tomatoes or an eight-ounce glass of tomato juice.) Nonfat pasta sauce is a good source of lycopene (cooking improves its absorption), as are strawberries. In one study, men who ate one-half cup of strawberries daily

The Arachidonic Acid Cascade

Arachidonic acid, an omega-6 fatty acid, is a double-edged sword. On the one hand, our health depends on it, as it is essential to the nervous and immune systems. On the other hand, too much arachidonic acid can be deadly. Unfortunately, Americans suffer from an overabundance, not a lack, of arachidonic acid. Excess arachidonic acid has been linked to the current epidemic of heart disease, degenerative diseases, and cancer in this country.

Inside the body, arachidonic acid is converted to powerful hormone-like molecules called *eicosanoids*. Two types of eicosanoids—called *prostaglandins* and *leukotrienes*—are derived from arachidonic acid. (Prostaglandins were first discovered in prostatic fluid.) Eicosanoids can either be inflammatory or anti-inflammatory. The types of eicosanoids that are found in fish *(prostaglandin E3)* are anti-inflammatory. The eicosanoids that are derived from arachidonic acid *(prostaglandin E2* and *series-4 leukotrienes)* are inflammatory. Arthritic joint pain and the throbbing pain of a headache are caused by inflammatory prostaglandins.

Arachidonic acid–derived eicosanoids cause more problems than just inflammation. To begin with, PGE2 eicosanoids enable prostate cancer cells to evade the immune system. PGE2 inactivates natural killer cells and cytotoxic T cells (immune cells that attach themselves to prostate cancer cells and kill them). This is particularly scary, since prostate cancer cells produce ten times as much PGE2 as normal prostate cells.

Series-4 leukotrienes, the other class of arachidonic acid–derived eicosanoids, are just as dangerous as PGE2. Series-4 leukotrienes by the name of *12-HETE* allow prostate cancer cells to form new blood vessels and invade surrounding tissues. Another class of series-4 leukotrienes, called *5-HETE,* stimulates prostate cancer growth and prevents prostate cancer cells from dying by preventing them from committing suicide.

Fortunately, the harmful effects of arachidonic acid can be blocked. A combination of nutritional, herbal, and pharmaceutical agents can interrupt the arachidonic acid cascade at three critical points by blocking three different enzymes:[13]

(continued)

Cell membrane phospholipids → phospholipase A2 → arachidonic acid
Arachidonic acid → cyclooxygenase 1 and 2 → prostaglandin E2 series
and
5- and 12-lipoxygenase → series 4 leukotrienes (5- and 12-HETE).

Phospholipase A2 Enzyme

This enzyme allows arachidonic acid to be mobilized from phospholipids (fats) in cell membranes. This conversion can be blocked by quercetin (page 96), vitamin E (page 135), licorice *(Glycyrrhiza glabra)*, turmeric *(Curcuma longa)* (page 139), and prescription corticosteroids.

5- and 12-Lipoxygenase Enzymes

This enzyme enables arachidonic acid to be converted to series four leucotrienes (5-HETE and 12-HETE). This conversion can be blocked by quercetin, vitamin E, fish oil (page 142), turmeric, red and yellow onions *(Allium cepa)*, garlic *(Allium sativum)* (page 139), and Indian frankencense *(Boswellia serrata)* (page 139).

Cyclooxygenase 1 and 2 Enzymes

These enzymes convert arachidonic acid to PGE2 eicosanoids. This conversion can be blocked by fish oil, ginger *(Zingiber officinale)*, black willow *(Saslix nigra)*, wintergreen *(Gaultheria procumbens)*, and nonsteroidal anti-inflammatory medications (aspirin and ibuprofen). Celebrex and Vioxx are two new anti-inflammatory prescription drugs that can suppress angiogenesis and prostate cancer cell growth by selectively blocking cyclooxygenase-2.

significantly lowered their risk of developing prostate cancer. Lycopene is also available in capsule form (see page 142).

• **Garlic.** Another suggestion is garlic; I recommend eating at least two cloves of fresh garlic daily or taking it in capsule form as a supplement (see page 139). Hint: Letting chopped garlic "rest" for ten minutes before cooking helps preserve the protective enzymes from being destroyed.

- **Cruciferous Vegetables.** Other vegetables recommended include cruciferous vegetables like cabbage, broccoli, Brussels sprouts, kale, and cauliflower, which contain a cancer-busting substance called *sulforaphane*. More than one hundred research studies report that eating cruciferous vegetables decreases the risk of cancer.
- **All Organic Produce.** I highly recommend that you try to eat as much organic produce as possible. More than four hundred different pesticides are sprayed on domestic food, a number of which can cause cancer. According to one survey, the produce most likely to be contaminated include domestic fresh peaches; domestic winter squash; apples, grapes, spinach, and pears (from both U.S. and foreign sources); and domestic green beans.

If you can't afford (or find) the additional cost of organic produce, be sure to thoroughly wash all produce and peel any vegetables to remove toxic pesticide residues.

Fiber

Dietary fiber (plant material that isn't digested) decreases the risk of prostate cancer by binding with and eliminating excess fat and hormones from the body. The National Cancer Institute recommends eating between 25 and 35 grams of fiber daily.

Sugar

As mentioned in previous chapters, limit or avoid refined sugar. If you must, satisfy your sweet tooth with dark chocolate, which is rich in antioxidants called proanthocyanadins. Also, try the herbal sweetener stevia *(Stevia rebaudiana);* available in most health food stores, stevia contains only one-tenth of a calorie per teaspoon. (Avoid use in pregnant or lactating women and in diabetic patients.)

Soy Protein

As recommended in the other chapters, incorporate soy protein in your diet. Derived from soybeans, and rich in cancer-fighting substances called *isoflavones* (most notably genistein), soy protein dramatically inhibits prostate cancer cell growth by blocking estrogen, inhibiting 5-alpha reductase, an enzyme that stimulates prostate cancer cell growth; by inhibiting tyrosine-specific protein kinase, which prostate cancer cells use as a growth factor; and by preventing the growth of new blood vessels cancer cells need to grow (angiogenesis).

There are many ways to incorporate soy into your diet. It is available in a variety of food items such as tempeh, tofu, soybeans (edamame), miso, soy milk, soy cheese, and soy flour. Try stir-frying tempeh or tofu with your favorite vegetables or substituting soy milk for dairy. There are also many cookbooks available on the subject. Genistein is also available in capsule form. Consume enough soy or supplement with capsules for at least 40 milligrams of genistein daily for prevention, and 80 milligrams daily for patients with prostate cancer. If cost isn't an issue, higher doses (as high as 200 milligrams or more) may be even more effective.

Diets That Prevent or Prolong Prostate Cancer

Studies have shown that vegetarian, Mediterranean, and macrobiotic diets reduce the risk of prostate cancer. A vegetarian diet is meat-free (including fish and chicken) but rich in whole grains, fruits, and vegetables. A Mediterranean diet is low in meat but high in whole grains, fruits, vegetables, and olive oil.

A macrobiotic diet is tailored to individual needs. Although it's primarily vegetarian, a macrobiotic diet allows some meat. According to one report, men with prostate cancer who ate a macrobiotic diet lived almost twice as long as those who didn't.[15] Although the study involved only a small group of men, the results are encouraging.

A unique blend of East and West, macrobiotics integrates a traditional diet of whole natural food with a good dose of spiritual philosophy. While most physicians are unaware of its attributes, macrobiotics is the most popular unconventional nutritional therapy used in the United States.

VITAMINS

Supplementing your diet with certain vitamins can also decrease the risk of prostate cancer. Much of the data on the cancer-protective benefits of vitamins are based on laboratory (cell culture) and animal studies. Even so, research suggests that vitamins can also benefit humans by decreasing carcinogen formation, improving detoxification of harmful substances, decreasing cancer cell growth, improving cellular communication, and controlling cellular differentiation and the expression of cancer.

Antioxidants work better in combination; therefore, I recommend taking a high-potency multivitamin. Even a high-potency multivitamin, though, may not contain the optimal amount of the cancer-preventive vitamins that are listed below. See how your vitamin stacks up by comparing its contents (listed on the bottle label) against the following list of vitamins. If your vitamin falls short, take additional vitamins to fill in the gaps. However, be careful not to exceed the maximum dosage.

Vitamin E

A number of studies have shown that vitamin E decreases prostate cancer incidence and mortality. Vitamin E (along with selenium) does this by preventing the accumulation of toxic by-products of hydrogen peroxide within the prostate. According to one widely quoted study, supplementing with as little as 50 international units (I.U.) of vitamin E daily reduces the incidence of prostate cancer by one third, and the death rate by 40 percent.[16] I recommend a brand of vitamin E that contains mixed tocopherols (see page 156). Take 400 I.U. once daily with meals. (Note: Excessive vitamin E [more than 3,000 I.U. daily] may be harmful. Vitamin E may also increase the risk of bleeding in patients taking blood thinners.)

Vitamin D

Vitamin D decreases the risk of prostate cancer by inhibiting cancer cell growth and promoting cancer cell death. I recommend supplementing with 400 I.U. of vitamin D twice daily. (Note: Excess vitamin D [above 1,000 I.U. daily] can be harmful.)

Vitamin A

Although most epidemiological studies fail to show a protective benefit against prostate cancer, vitamin A is crucial for cell growth and differentiation. In animal studies, vitamin A can prevent the induction and promotion of cancer, and in laboratory tests it can even reverse malignant changes in prostate cancer cells. I recommend supplementing with 10,000 I.U. once daily. (Note: Excessive vitamin A [daily doses above 50,000 I.U.] may be harmful.)

Beta-carotene

Brightly colored vegetables are a rich source of the provitamin beta-carotene. (It is called a provitamin because the body converts it to another vitamin—vitamin A.) The history of beta-carotene and prostate cancer prevention is controversial.

Although reports vary, according to several studies, low levels of beta-carotene pose a significant risk for prostate cancer. Even though another highly publicized study found an increased risk of prostate cancer in smokers who supplemented with beta-carotene (but not in smokers who supplemented with vitamin E in addition to beta-carotene), other studies report no increased risk. In fact, data from the Physicians' Health Study suggest that men who supplement with 50,000 I.U. of beta-carotene daily have a significantly lower risk of developing prostate cancer (especially if they have a low beta-carotene level).[17] Therefore, I tell patients that the amount of beta-carotene typically found in a high-potency vitamin (25,000 I.U.) is not only safe but also may even prevent prostate cancer.

Vitamin C

Although not specific for prostate cancer, the vast majority of more than ninety epidemiological studies have found that vitamin C exerts a significant protective effect against cancer. In laboratory studies, vitamin C inhibits prostate cancer. I recommend taking at least one gram of vitamin C in divided doses daily. Vitamin C is extremely safe, even at high doses.

Although taking high doses of vitamin C is not specific for prostate cancer, it may improve the quality of life and survival of cancer patients. According to Nobel laureate Linus Pauling, cancer patients who supplemented their diets with at least 10 grams of vitamin C daily (in divided doses) lived longer and felt better.

HERBS

Scientific research suggests that the herbs listed below, although not specific for prostate cancer, may help prevent the initiation, promotion, and progression stages of prostate cancer.

As a general measure, I tell *all* of my male patients to drink green tea or take a green tea extract. However, if you have prostate cancer, or if there is a strong family history of prostate cancer, I recommend taking all of the following herbs (except PC-SPES, which should be taken only under medical supervision). If finances are an issue, select a few herbs that you can afford (I've listed the herbs in the order of preference).

Green Tea *(Camellia sinensis)*

According to researchers at the University of Chicago, green tea not only inhibits the growth of prostate cancer cells (in animals), but also reduces the size of existing tumors.[18] Green tea is rich in a group of flavonoid antioxidants called *catechins*. One of these catechins—*epigallocatechin gallate* (EGCG)—has two hundred times the antioxidant power of vitamin E. Furthermore, EGCG kills hormone-insensitive prostate cancer cells. Researchers theorize that green tea prevents cancer by preventing DNA strand breaks, inhibiting cell proliferation, decreasing the contact of carcinogens with cells, blocking cancer initiation, and slowing cancer progression. Since the protective benefit of green tea is dose dependent, I recommend taking 500 milligrams of an herbal extract (standardized to contain 80 percent total polyphenol and 55 percent EGCG) once daily for prevention and twice daily for men with prostate cancer.

Stinging Nettle *(Urtica dioica)*

Stinging nettle root may prevent prostate cancer by inhibiting the binding of sex-hormone-binding globulin (SHBG) to the prostate cell membrane. In addition, nettles prevent prostate cancer by blocking the conversion of androgens to estrogens (a process known as *aromatization*), and by inhibiting the biosynthesis of arachidonic acid metabolites that stimulate prostate cancer cell growth and progression. (For more information, see page 55.)

The normal daily dose is three to six grams, taken as a tablet or capsule containing 600 to 1,200 milligrams of a 5:1 dry extract, or 120 milligrams twice daily of a 10:1 extract (standardized for amino acid content). There are no known contraindications, drug interactions, or significant side effects.

Milk Thistle *(Silybum marianum)*

Rich in antioxidant flavonoids known as silymarin, an extract of milk thistle seeds has been shown to inhibit prostate cancer initiation, promotion, and progression. Researchers report that milk thistle works by altering signaling molecules and adaptor proteins affecting epidermal growth factor receptor (a potent stimulus of cell growth). As a result, prostate cancer cells, even androgen-resistant prostate cancer cells (the most dangerous kind), stop growing.[19]

Since the protective effect of milk thistle is dose dependent, I recommend 250 milligrams four times daily with food. Buy a standardized extract that contains 70 percent silymarin complex. There are no known contraindications, drug interactions, or side effects.

Cernilton

In addition to treating BPH and prostatitis, Cernilton inhibits the growth of prostate cancer. The recommended dosage varies according to the product. Follow the instructions on the bottle. (See pages 54 and 85 in Chapters 2 and 3 for additional information on Cernilton.)

Turmeric *(Curcuma longa)*

A potent antioxidant, turmeric (the major ingredient of curry powder) may inhibit prostate cancer by blocking the conversion of arachidonic acid to PGE2 and 5-HETE, inducing apoptosis, and regulating the tumor suppressor gene *p53*.[20] The recommended dose is 400 to 600 milligrams, three times daily. There are no side effects or drug interactions. The only contraindication is obstruction of the bile passages.

Indian Frankincense *(Boswellia serrata)*

Derived from the gum resin of a tree native to India, Indian frankincense may prevent prostate cancer by inhibiting the conversion of arachidonic acid to 5-HETE.[21] The recommended dose is 400 milligrams of a standardized extract (containing 60 percent boswellic acid), taken three times daily. There are no significant side effects.

Pygeum *(Prunus africana)*

Pygeum is derived from the bark of the African plum tree. Although the exact mechanism of action is unknown, pygeum may prevent prostate cancer by blocking the conversion of arachidonic acid to 5-HETE, reducing serum prolactin levels and preventing prostate cell proliferation.[22] (See page 52 for more information on recommended dosage.)

Saw Palmetto *(Serenoa repens)*

Best known as an effective treatment for prostate enlargement, saw palmetto may also prevent prostate cancer. There are no known significant side effects, drug interactions, or contraindications. (See page 50 for more information.)

Garlic *(Allium sativum)*

Since fresh garlic costs only pennies a day, I've listed the more expensive garlic supplements last on the list. Both fresh garlic and garlic supplements prevent prostate cancer by interfering with its initiation and promotion phases and by blocking arachidonic acid metabolism.[24] The quality of garlic supplements varies. Therefore, choose one that is standardized for its allicin content (it should contain at least 4,000 *micro*grams of allicin). Take 4,000 *milli*grams of garlic equivalent (equal to two cloves of fresh garlic) daily. There are no known drug interactions or contraindications; however, garlic can occasionally cause gastrointestinal symptoms or allergic reactions. Furthermore, excessive garlic can increase the risk of bleeding in patients that take blood thinners.

PC-SPES

PC-SPES is the brand name for a product made by BotanicLab. *PC* stands for prostate cancer; *spes* is latin for hope. It contains eight different Chinese herbs including licorice, chrysanthemum, and saw palmetto. PC-SPES stops prostate cancer cell growth by inducing apoptosis and causing differentiation (reduction or reversal of cancer activity). Scientific research has shown that PC-SPES kills prostate cancer cells in men with hormone-sensitive and hormone-resistant prostate cancer.

Columbia University researchers treated a group of thirty-three men with PC-SPES. They reported that within two months of starting PC-SPES, 87 percent of the men experienced a drop in their PSA levels, and the improvement lasted for at least six months in 78 percent of the men.[25] Other researchers at University of California at San Francisco reported similar findings.[26] Among a group of seventy men who were treated with PC-SPES, the PSA level fell by more than 50 percent in the 100 percent of patients who had androgen-dependent tumors and in 54 percent of men with androgen-independent cancers. Furthermore, the researchers noted that metastatic bone lesions shrank in a number of the men who received PC-SPES.

Although effective, PC-SPES can cause a number of side effects, some of which are serious. These side effects include skin rash, nausea, impotence, breast tenderness, fluid retention, blood clots, and pulmonary embolus (blood clots that travel to the lungs). Unfortunately, since the manufacturer doesn't list these potentially dangerous side effects on the product label, most patients are unaware of them. PC-SPES should be taken only by men with biopsy-proven prostate cancer who are under the supervision of a urologist or oncologist. Dosage depends on the individual, but the usual dose is two to three 320-milligram capsules taken three times daily.

SUPPLEMENTS

A variety of safe and cost-effective supplements plays a vital role in decreasing the incidence and modulating the promotion and progression of prostate cancer. Scientific studies suggest that the following supplements may possibly decrease the incidence, promotion, and progression of prostate cancer:

Selenium

According to a landmark study reported in the *Journal of the American Medical Association,* men who supplemented their diet with the trace element selenium reduced their risk of prostate cancer by two-thirds.[27] Selenium also decreased the promotion and progression of prostate cancer. Furthermore, selenium also improves immune function and decreases the absorption of toxic metals (such as cadmium) that can increase the risk of developing prostate cancer.

Although plants absorb selenium from the soil, food that is grown in selenium-deficient soil won't contain sufficient amounts of this cancer-protective micronutrient. This applies to the following states and regions of the United States: Pennsylvania, Ohio, the eastern two-thirds of Washington State and Oregon, northern California, the Atlantic Coastal Plain, and the upper Mississippi River valley. In contrast, the northern Great Plains is rich in selenium.

If you live in a selenium-deficient area of the United States, supplement your diet with 200 micrograms of yeast-derived selenium daily. If you are allergic to yeast, take 200 micrograms of selenomethionine or selenocysteine (contained in selenoglutathione or selenodiglutathione preparations) daily. *Be sure to take into account the amount of selenium already contained in your multivitamin.*

If you live in a selenium-rich region, or if you are unsure, ask your doctor to check your selenium level (it should be around 200 micrograms per milliliter). Incidentally, the earlier in life selenium is started, the greater the protective benefits. (Note: Excess selenium [usually above 600 micrograms daily] may be toxic.)

Genistein

As mentioned earlier, the isoflavone genistein found in soy decreases the incidence, growth, and spead of prostate cancer (see page 134).

Lycopene

For those men who can't tolerate eating tomatoes, they can still obtain the cancer-preventive benefits of tomatoes (see page 132) by taking supplemental lycopene. Take a 10-milligram oil-based lycopene capsule twice daily with meals for prevention, or three times daily if there is a family history of prostate cancer or if prostate cancer is present.

Fish Oil

Rich in an essential omega-3 fatty acid called *eicosapentaenoic acid (EPA)*, fish oil decreases the risk of prostate cancer by suppressing arachidonic acid formation. I recommend selecting a product that is standardized for EPA (and assayed to exclude mercury contamination).

Take up to six grams a day with meals in conjunction with gamma linolenic acid (GLA) (see below). Strive for a ratio of 5:1 EPA to GLA. (Note: Use only under a doctor's supervision if you are taking a blood thinner.)

Black Currant, Borage, or Primrose Oil

Rich in an omega-6 fatty acid called *gamma linolenic acid (GLA)*, these three oils block prostate cell growth by blocking the production of a potent growth factor called urokinase-type plasminogen activator.[28] Of the three oils, borage oil is the most cost effective and contains the most GLA. Take up to one and a half grams of borage oil (standardized for GLA) daily with meals.

Docosahexaenoic acid *(DHA)*

Not to be confused with DHEA (see page 144), DHA is an omega-3 fatty acid that is manufactured from algae. DHA is available in 100- and 200-milligram capsules (brand name Neuromins). Although not proven, 1,000 milligrams taken daily in divided doses may inhibit prostate cancer.[29]

Zinc

Researchers have recently discovered that the essential micronutrient zinc, while not specific for prostate cancer, inhibits the growth of prostate cancer cells and enhances apoptosis.[30] Studies show that marginal zinc deficiency is common, especially among the elderly. Therefore, I recommend supplementing with 30 to 60 milligrams of zinc daily (taking into account the amount of zinc already in your multivitamin). (See page 95 for more information on zinc.) (Note: Taking excessive zinc [greater than 150 milligrams daily] depresses copper levels, impairs immune function, and interferes with the action of selenium. In addition, calcium and iron interfere with zinc absorption, so don't take them together.)

Supplements That Should be Taken Only Under Certain Circumstances

Patients who have androgen-resistant cancer, or those men with an increased risk for metastatic disease (if the PSA is greater than 20, the Gleason score is over 7, or the pathology report from surgery shows that the prostate cancer has spread locally beyond the prostate) may slow the progression of their cancer by taking the following supplements:

- **Melatonin.** Melatonin, a hormone made in the brain by the pineal gland, directly and indirectly inhibits the growth of prostate cancer cells. It does this by decreasing the production of prolactin and IGF-1, stimulating the anti-tumor immune system, and causing differentiation of cancer cells. According to one study, over half of the patients with hormone-resistant prostate cancer taking melatonin (20 milligrams at bedtime) had their hormone sensitivity restored![31] (Taking supplemental melatonin doesn't interfere with the brain's normal production of melatonin.) Research has also shown that melatonin can enhance chemotherapy effectiveness. Patients with androgen-resistant prostate cancer may wish to consider taking 20 milligrams of melatonin one hour before bedtime. (Note: Although melatonin doesn't cause any serious side effects, it can cause drowsiness.)

- **Modified Citrus Pectin.** Derived from specially treated citrus fruit fiber (to make it more absorbable), modified citrus pectin slows PSA doubling time and inhibits prostate cancer metastases.[32] Although the use of modified citrus pectin is experimental, patients at risk for developing metastatic prostate cancer may consider taking five grams of powder (Pecta-Sol brand by EcoNugenics) mixed in water or juice three times daily.
- **High Doses of Zinc.** On page 143, I recommended zinc supplements as a possible prevention for prostate cancer, but in small doses of no more 60 mg per day. However, if you have prostate cancer, high doses of zinc (50 milligrams taken three times daily) can kill prostate cancer cells by depriving them of copper. Copper suppresses prostate cancer cell growth and prevents angiogenesis. Within four to six months of taking 150 mg of zinc daily, the copper level falls by 70 to 90 percent. The only side effect appears to be a mild anemia.[33] (Note: High doses of zinc should be taken only under medical supervision.)

Supplements That Should Be Avoided

Both DHEA (dehydroepiandrosterone) and chondroitin sulfate should be avoided if you have prostate cancer. DHEA has been hyped as a way to prevent everything from aging to cancer, but it can make prostate cancer grow faster by boosting serum IGF-1 levels.

Chondroitin sulfate is popular for treating osteoarthritis. Three recent studies have suggested that there may be a link between chondroitin sulfate and the spread of prostate cancer.[34] Although the results are preliminary, men with prostate cancer (or a strong family history of prostate cancer) should avoid chondroitin sulfate pending further studies.

Natural Therapies to Aid
Cancer Treatment

Although radiation therapy (RT) and chemotherapy (CT) may halt prostate cancer's relentless progress, the accompanying side effects often leave patients wondering if the cure is worse than the disease. The following natural remedies can reduce the side effects of RT and CT, which often include hair loss, anemia, impaired fertility, nausea, diarrhea, loss of appetite, and malnutrition. Also, some of these remedies can help enhance the effectiveness of these treatments. Furthermore, I'll also offer natural remedies for some of the other side effects caused by androgen-deprivation therapy, which include hot flashes, osteoporosis, and liver damage.

LIFESTYLE CHANGES

The lifestyle changes discussed elsewhere in this chapter also apply here. Follow the diet advice beginning on page 47 in Chapter 2 and page 75 in Chapter 3. In addition to this advice, make sure you have enough protein (1 to 2 grams per kilogram [2.2 lbs.] of body weight). Reducing stress and massage therapy are also effective in reducing side effects. I also recommend that you explore traditional Chinese medicine techniques, such as acupuncture, and try employing mind-body techniques like the Healing Imagery exercise on page 83. (Note: Substitute the words *prostate cancer* for *prostatitis*). These steps will all help to alleviate the side effects of RT and CT and help to improve their overall effectiveness.

VITAMINS AND SUPPLEMENTS

Despite the potential benefits, some physicians advise against taking antioxidant vitamins and supplements during RT and CT. They believe that taking antioxidant vitamins, herbs, or supplements during RT and CT may prevent these treatments from effectively doing their job (killing cancer cells). They worry that taking antioxidants may exchange fewer acute side effects for a less effective therapy. (Note: Certain chemotherapy drugs are affected more than others by antioxidants.)

Other experts argue that antioxidants can be safely taken during RT and CT. In fact, according to one research team, there are only three documented examples in which an antioxidant has been shown to decrease the effectiveness of radiation or chemotherapy *in vivo* (in humans).

Furthermore, they claim that the vast majority of animal and human research studies has shown that antioxidants enhance the effectiveness or have a neutral effect on cancer therapies.[35]

Until there are conclusive data, I recommend checking with your oncologist before taking multivitamins or supplements during chemotherapy or radiation therapy. However, you can still safely eat plenty of antioxidant-containing fruits and vegetables. In addition to causing free-radical damage, RT and CT deplete the body of vitamins. Although antioxidants made by the body, and those obtained from the diet, combat the free radicals that are generated by RT and CT, taking a high-potency multivitamin offers additional protection.

Vitamins can also prevent other radiation-induced complications. For instance, investigators have discovered that 400 I.U. of vitamin E plus 400 milligrams of pentoxifylline (brand name Trental, a prescription medication that improves blood flow) taken twice daily can reverse radiation-induced bladder fibrosis (scarring).[36]

Taking the following supplements (either singly or in combination), including selenium (see page 141) and green tea (see page 137) can minimize some of the devastating side effects that can result from radiation therapy and chemotherapy:

Shiitake Mushroom *(Lentinula edodes)*
According to one report, patients who consumed a shiitake mushroom extract in conjunction with radiation therapy and chemotherapy had significantly fewer side effects.[37] It also increase the effectiveness of these treatments. Take 150 milligrams of dried extract or eat four cooked mushrooms daily.

Maitake Mushroom *(Grifola)*
The D-fraction of a maitake mushroom enhances the immune system and minimizes side effects of chemotherapy.[38] Purchase an extract that is standardized for the D-fraction. Take one-half to one milligram per kilogram daily between meals.

Reishi Mushroom *(Ganoderma lucidum)*

Taking an extract of reishi mushrooms can minimize bone marrow suppression and fatigue due to radiation therapy and chemotherapy.[39]

On an empty stomach, take a total daily dose of five to ten grams of dried fruit body, or an equivalent amount of extract.

N-Acetyl-Cysteine

A precursor to glutathione (a key antioxidant that is used by the liver to detoxify toxins), N-acetyl-cysteine decreases the side effects of hemorrhagic cysititis (bloody urine) caused by cyclophosphamide (a common cancer drug) and doxorubicin-induced heart damage.[40] Use 600 milligrams of N-acetyl-cysteine daily on an empty stomach.

L-Glutamine

Used selectively by the intestinal cells as fuel, the amino acid L-glutamine protects against radiation-induced damage to the intestinal lining (particularly diarrhea).[41] Take three grams of L-glutamine powder three times daily on an empty stomach.

Pectin Fiber

A soluble fiber derived from fruit, pectin minimizes intestinal cell damage caused by a chemotherapy drug called methotrexate.[42] Take between five and ten grams daily in divided doses before meals.

Ginkgo Biloba

Highly regarded for its positive effect on the vascular system, *Ginkgo biloba* also reduces doxorubicin-induced side effects.[43] It also enhances the effectiveness of RT and CT. Take 80 milligrams of an extract (standardized to contain 24 percent ginkgo heterosides) three times daily.

Coenzyme Q_{10}

Although pricey, the potent antioxidant coenzyme Q_{10} inhibits doxorubicin-induced cardiac damage, prevents free-radical damage caused by lipid peroxidation, and spares vitamin E from oxidative degradation.[44] Take at least 50 milligrams of coenzyme Q_{10} daily.

Astragalus *(Astragalus membranaceus)*

According to a team of American and Chinese researchers, the "F-fraction" of this tonic herb also improves the effectiveness of interleukin-2 used in CT.[45] This means that a lesser amount of this toxic agent may achieve the same results. Take one capsule three times daily. (Note: Astragalus may contain excess selenium. Therefore, don't take supplemental selenium in addition to astragalus.)

Cloud Mushroom *(Coriolus versicolor)*

According to Japanese researchers, cloud mushroom increases life span when it's taken in conjunction with RT and CT.[46] Take one gram three times daily.

PREVENTING SECONDARY
MALIGNANCIES DUE TO RT AND CT

Radiation therapy and chemotherapy can damage the genetic information (DNA) in normal cells. Consequently, these cancer therapies can actually *cause* cancer.

Even though the structures around the prostate (such as the bladder and rectum) are shielded against the harmful effects of radiation, they are still caught in the cross fire of radiation beams. Although the radiation-induced changes aren't immediately apparent, cancer can develop years later.

As mentioned earlier, bladder cancer is the most common type of cancer that develops following external beam irradiation to the prostate. In addition to the previous advice on lifestyle and diet, scientific research has shown that the following nutritional measures reduce the risk of bladder cancer:

- Vitamins (40,000 I.U. vitamin A; 100 mg vitamin B_6; 2,000 mg vitamin C; 400 I.U. vitamin E; 90 mg zinc)[47]

- At least 64 ounces of water daily[48]
- Green tea (see page 137)[49]
- *Lactobacillus casei* (see page 97)[50]

SIDE EFFECTS OF ANDROGEN-DEPRIVATION THERAPY

Hot flashes and osteoporosis are two common side effects of androgen-deprivation therapy (male hormone withdrawal). Men treated in this fashion often complain that these two conditions make their lives miserable. Fortunately, prescription drugs and a variety of natural remedies can reduce the incidence and severity of these common side effects.

Natural therapies can also prevent liver damage, particularly hepatitis (liver inflammation)—a rare but potentially fatal complication of androgen-deprivation therapy.

Hot Flashes

When male hormone is removed, most men experience hot flashes. Similar to the hot flashes women experience during menopause, men experience sudden skin flushing accompanied by profuse sweating. Although anecdotal (based on experience), I have found that eating soy protein and following the lifestyle suggestions found throughout this book can minimize these flashes. In addition, take a dropperful (forty drops) of a standardized liquid extract or one capsule of dried extract of the following herbs twice daily: chasteberry *(Vitex agnus-castus)*, dong quai *(Angelica sinensis)*, and damiana *(Turnera diffusa)*. Add 400 mg of vitamin E and 50 mg of vitamin B complex twice a day to your multivitamin. Finally, acupuncture can eliminate hot flashes in men.

Osteoporosis

The moment men are started on androgen-deprivation therapy, they begin losing bone mass. Complications of bone loss include bone pain and a greater risk of bone fractures. In addition to prescription drugs, try exercise, diet changes, and soy protein, and supplement with calcium-magnesium citrate (containing 1,000 milligrams of calcium and 500 to 1,000 milligrams of magnesium) and ipriflavone (an isoflavone derivative), 200 mg three times daily.

Hepatitis

Hepatitis is a rare but dangerous side effect of oral anti-androgen therapy. Men taking these two drugs should avoid substances that can impair liver function (such as alcoholic beverages and acetaminophen). Follow the previous advice on multivitamins, vitamins E and C, milk thistle, and fruits and vegetables. In addition, the following natural therapies may prevent drug-induced liver damage:[51]

- **Alpha-lipoic acid.** This coenzyme works with an antioxidant called glutathione to protect the liver. Take one 300-milligram capsule twice daily.
- **N-acetyl-L-cysteine.** This antioxidant amino acid restores and maintains glutathione levels in the liver. Take one 600-milligram capsule three times daily.
- **Pycnogenol** (Pinus pinaster). Derived from pine bark, pycnogenol contains bioflavonoids (antioxidants) that support liver function. Take 50 milligrams daily.

How to Become a Cancer Survivor

While it's not always possible to achieve a cure, it is possible to improve the quality of life and prolong the survival of men with prostate cancer. In addition to lifestyle changes, proper diet (especially a macrobiotic diet), vitamins, and supplements, scientific research has proven that mind-body medicine can have an enormous impact on prolonging the survival of cancer patients.

GROUP THERAPY

There is abundant evidence that psychosocial interventions improve the quality of life of cancer patients. They also improve the survival of men with prostate cancer.

Researchers compared the survival and quality of life among twenty-nine men with early-stage prostate cancer.[52] Men who attended at least five out of six specially designed support group meetings were compared against a matched group of sixty-five men who didn't attend these meetings.

Attendees at the support meetings discussed seven different topics: (1) the effect of one's beliefs, feelings, and attitudes on health; (2) mental relaxation and imagery techniques; (3) nutrition and exercise; (4) stress management; (5) self-esteem and spirituality; (6) receptive imagery/intuition and problem solving; and (7) creating a personal health plan/goal setting. The men attending the meetings also were given an audiotape on guided imagery and were encouraged to read several books on the same topic.

The results were astounding. The treatment group not only enjoyed a better quality of life but also lived twice as long as the control group.

OTHER ALTERNATIVE MEDICINE THERAPIES

While this chapter focuses on *allopathic* (Western) medicine, other healing traditions such as naturopathic medicine, Ayurvedic medicine, and traditional Chinese medicine approach prostate cancer differently than does Western medicine. Furthermore, physicians who practice in alternative medicine cancer clinics in this country and abroad treat prostate cancer differently than do their mainstream medical colleagues. Although these and other alternative therapies for prostate cancer deserve further study, their discussion is beyond the scope of this book.

TRAITS OF CANCER SURVIVORS

As with child rearing, an instruction manual doesn't come with the diagnosis of cancer. There is a book, though, that is helpful in this regard. *Choices in Healing,* written by Michael Lerner, Ph.D., provides patients with a blueprint that outlines how to cope with cancer. Based on more than ten years of painstaking research, Lerner's book explores the controversies between orthodox and alternative treatments for cancer in terms that a nonprofessional can understand. Drawing on reliable scientific studies, Lerner makes a convincing argument for treating cancer with a blend of the best of conventional and alternative therapies. He also offers advice on how to become a "cancer survivor."

Lerner explains that certain traits appear to offer cancer patients a survival advantage. One of these traits is regarding illness (cancer) as a gift—as a turning point in their lives. Appreciating the wisdom of this concept—cancer as a gift—requires much soul-searching. For some, the connection is easy to see—they've been cured of their cancers. For others, especially those with incurable disease, the blessing may elude them.

Whether cancer is seen as a blessing or not, I encourage my patients to reflect on what really matters in their lives and "don't sweat the small stuff." In addition, like Lerner, I've also found that cancer survivors exhibit the following traits:

- not taking "no" for an answer
- actively searching for help
- seeking out others who have been healed from their type of cancer
- forming constructive partnerships with health professionals
- finding a purpose in life
- cultivating self-acceptance
- avoiding constant thoughts about undesirable developments
- cultivating a balanced optimism
- not hesitating to make radical life changes

Finally, Lerner discusses the difference between a cure and healing. A cure is the complete absence of disease for the rest of one's life. Doctors hope to bring a cure to men whom they treat for prostate cancer. Unfortunately, this is not always possible. Healing, on the other hand, is *always* possible. Healing is an inner process that takes place on an emotional, mental, and spiritual level.

As a tribute to the millions of men with prostate cancer, I presented a speech titled "Spirituality and Prostate Cancer" at the American Holistic Medical Association's twenty-third national convention. In my speech, I described the three phases of a hero's quest (accepting the call, the journey, and enlightenment) and encouraged all men with prostate cancer to embark on such a journey. The text of my speech is available on my website (www.urolmd.com) under the heading "Mind/Body/Spirit Medicine."

Conclusion

Most men, if they live long enough, will develop prostate cancer. Fortunately, most of these men won't die because of prostate cancer. Nevertheless, harmful dietary, environmental, and lifestyle choices increase the likelihood of dying from prostate cancer. Conversely, substituting healthy choices for unhealthy ones dramatically reduces the risk of developing and dying from prostate cancer. For instance, the natural therapies listed in this chapter can prevent or alter the initiation, promotion, and progression stages of prostate cancer.

PSA screening has revolutionized the early diagnosis of prostate cancer. Consequently, more men than ever before are being cured of prostate cancer. Even so, once prostate cancer has spread beyond the prostate, a cure isn't always possible. In this situation, aggressive therapies are needed to halt its progress. Unfortunately, these drastic measures often result in a number of unpleasant side effects.

Scientific research has shown that natural remedies can soften the blow of treatment-related side effects. In addition, natural remedies can enhance the effectiveness of many conventional cancer therapies. Finally, natural remedies can even improve the quality of life and survival of men with prostate cancer.

5

Conclusion

The theme for this book is prevention. Throughout, I've equipped you with the knowledge you need to maintain a healthy prostate. As you've learned, BPH and prostate cancer don't occur overnight; they develop over decades as a consequence of environmental, dietary, lifestyle, and genetic influences. Although the genetic make-up of the prostate can't be altered, the other three influences *can be*. Healthy choices in each of these three categories can decrease the risk of developing prostate disease, whereas unhealthy choices have the opposite effect. Remarkably, healthy choices can also favorably influence the genetic expression of prostate disease.

Although urologists regard prostatitis as the black sheep of the prostate family of diseases, the comprehensive program for prostatitis outlined in this book is an effective antidote for even the most stubborn case of prostatitis.

Now that you are armed with all this information, use it to take charge of your health. Explore the options available to you. As you have learned, surgery and medication are no longer your only choices. You have alternatives. Good prostate health can be yours.

Appendix A

A Brief Overview of Nutritional Supplements

Government-sponsored studies have shown that 50 percent of the American population have marginal nutrient deficiencies and that only 20 percent of individuals consume the minimum recommended daily dietary allowance of nutrients. Furthermore, prescription drugs compound the problem by interfering with the absorption or utilization of precious vitamins and minerals. Therefore, in addition to eating a well-balanced diet, I recommend taking a daily multivitamin.

VITAMINS AND MINERALS

Vitamins are essential organic compounds that our bodies use for normal metabolic function. (The Latin word *vita* means "life.") Vitamins are called *essential,* because bodies can't manufacture most of them. They're also called *micronutrients,* because they're needed only in small amounts. Before vitamins can be utilized, though, the body must first convert them into another substance called a *coenzyme.* Coenzymes make enzymes work better. Enzymes are substances that catalyze chemical reactions in the body.

Like vitamins, minerals are micronutrients that are essential for proper health. Eighteen different minerals play a role in human physiology. Minerals are also needed for proper bone growth, muscle contractions, and nerve function. Vitamins and minerals form a buddy system: As coenzymes, they help each other initiate or facilitate biochemical reactions, which explains why multivitamins contain a mixture of both products.

TYPES

Vitamins are either *water-soluble* or *fat-soluble.* As their name implies, water-soluble vitamins dissolve in water. The B vitamins and vitamin C make up the family of water-soluble vitamins. Water-soluble vitamins can't be stored (they're excreted in the urine over a period of one to four days). Therefore, water-soluble vitamins must be taken daily. As a rule, since water-soluble vitamins don't accumulate in the body, they have a wide safety range and are rarely toxic.

Fat-soluble vitamins (which include vitamins D, E, A, and K) are stored in adipose tissue (body fat) and the liver. Therefore, it's possible to get an overdose of fat-soluble vitamins. Just the same, if taken as directed, fat-soluble vitamins rarely cause serious side effects, and, if they occur, most are reversible once the vitamins are stopped.

Although vitamins are available in a variety of shapes, sizes, and formulations, they're all well absorbed and utilized as long as they're made by a reputable company (see the discussion below) and taken as directed. (As a general rule, vitamins should be taken with food.)

In natural foods, vitamins are bound to proteins, lipids (fat), carbohydrates, and bioflavonoids (compounds that are found in green plants). Vitamins that are derived from natural foods are called *natural vitamins.* In contrast, synthetic vitamins are made in the laboratory from isolated chemicals that mirror natural vitamins. However, the difference between the two types of vitamins matters only if the natural form is better absorbed or utilized than the synthetic form. With the exception of vitamin E, natural and synthetic vitamins work equally well. (Natural vitamin E [mixed tocopherols] works better.)

Minerals are divided into two groups: major minerals and minor (trace) minerals. The body needs at least 100 milligrams (one milligram equals one-thousandth of a gram) of the major minerals (calcium, magnesium, sodium, potassium, and phosphorus) daily. In contrast, the body needs only microgram (one microgram equals one-millionth of a gram) amounts of trace elements (such as selenium) daily.

The best way to ensure that you get a sufficient amount of minerals is to eat plenty of fresh vegetables. Just the same, the following factors influence mineral intake: individual dietary habits; mineral content of the soil; degree of intestinal absorption; and influence of other minerals. Binding minerals to a protein in the middle of a larger molecule, a process called *chelation,* enhances mineral absorption. For example, zinc picolinate, one of the best-absorbed zinc supplements, is formulated by chelating zinc to an organic salt called "picolinate."

As a rule, minerals are also better absorbed when they are taken with food. There are exceptions to the rule, though. For instance, fiber supplements decrease mineral absorption; hence, they should not be taken together. In addition to fiber, calcium absorption is impaired by excess dietary fat, caffeine, and alcohol. (Try taking calcium at bedtime, since it's not only better absorbed, but also promotes sleep.) Finally, too much calcium adversely affects magnesium absorption; therefore, choose a calcium supplement that is balanced in a 1:1 or 2:1 ratio with magnesium.

SAFETY

Contrary to popular belief, vitamins have a wide safety range. Scientific studies have shown that high doses of individual vitamins, particularly water-soluble vitamins, can be safely given to prevent or treat certain conditions without any associated serious side effects. Nevertheless, vitamins and minerals can affect the absorption or action of prescription medication, and high doses of fat-soluble vitamins (in excess of the amount contained in a multivitamin) can cause harmful side effects.

Although minerals also have a wide safety range, when taken in excessive amounts, they too can cause harmful side effects. For instance, taking more than 100 mg of zinc daily can cause a copper deficiency, and taking more than 900 mg of selenium daily can be toxic. Furthermore, minerals can interfere with the absorption of certain antibiotics and other medications. For instance, zinc and calcium adversely affect the absorption of quinilone antibiotics (e.g., Cipro). *Therefore, if you take prescription medication, check with your physician before taking supplemental minerals or vitamins.*

Dietary Supplement

Serving size: *six capsules*

SIX CAPSULES CONTAIN:		% **DV**
Vitamin C:	1,200 mg	1,333%
Vitamin E:	400 IU	1,818%
Selenium:	200 mcg	363%
Vanadium:	50 mcg	*
Bromelain:	25 mg	*
L-cysteine:	200 mg	*

*Daily value not established

Other ingredients: *cellulose and magnesium stearate*

Best if used by: *January 2002*

HOW TO READ A VITAMIN LABEL

As a final measure, let me teach you how to read a vitamin label. Items in bold type are discussed in further detail.

Translated, here's what the highlighted terms in the label mean:

- **Serving size** is the unit of measure (number of capsules, in this case) that must be taken to yield the daily amount specified on the label.
- **DV** stands for "Daily Value," or the recommended daily amount.
- **1,333%** indicates that the 1,200 mg of vitamin C contained in a serving (six tablets) is 13.33 times (or 1,333%) the recommended

daily amount of vitamin C (90 milligrams for nonsmoking men). Although high-potency multivitamins contain vitamin concentrations that are hundreds or even thousands of times greater than the DV, don't be alarmed—they're safe to take. The DV was established to prevent nutritional disease, not to promote optimal health.

- The abbreviation **mg** stands for *milli*gram.
- The abbreviation **mcg** stands for *micro*gram.
- Many vitamin supplements contain ingredients that don't have an established daily requirement. These items include certain trace elements (such as **vanadium**), digestive enzymes, and amino acids. Digestive enzymes (chemicals that promote digestion) are identified by their word endings: Words that end in "ain" (such as **bromelain**—a digestive enzyme made from pineapple) or "ase" (such as lipase—a digestive pancreatic enzyme) are digestive enzymes. (The bottle should state whether the enzymes are derived from plant or animal sources.) Amino acids (the building blocks of proteins) are identified by a "L" or "DL" before their name—for example, **L-cysteine.**
- **Other ingredients:** Read this section carefully. Supplements often contain other ingredients that are best avoided, such as artificial coloring, preservatives, flavorings, corn, soy protein, wheat gluten, sugar, yeast, and dairy products. These "fillers" can cause an allergic reaction in susceptible individuals.
- **Best if used by:** Signifies the expiration date.

RECOMMENDED BRANDS

I recommend protecting yourself by purchasing vitamins from companies that conform to *good manufacturing practices*. This is, give your business to a company that lists all of the ingredients on the bottle label or package insert; assays their products for purity and batch-to-batch consistency; doesn't make false claims; lists an expiration date on their products;

conforms to industry standards of excellence; and provides a certificate of analysis upon request.

Based on my research and experience, I have become familiar with the following companies, which manufacture *over-the-counter brands* that I trust: Enzymatic Therapies, Nutricology, Ethical Nutrients, Solgar, Jarrow Formulas, Solaray, Nature's Way, Nature's Plus, Source Naturals, Life Extension Foundation, and Twin Labs.

Similarly, companies that manufacture *"professional brands only"* (available only through pharmacies or health professionals) that I trust include: PhytoPharmica, Metagenics, Biotics Research, Tyler Encapsulations, CVR/Ecological Formulas, Thorne Research, ARG/Allergy Research Group, Pure Encapsulations, Murdock Madaus Schwabe (MMS Pro), Douglas Laboratories, Priority One, and American Biotics.

Appendix B
A Brief Overview of Herbal Supplements

Herbs have been used for millennia to promote wellness and treat disease. Although herbs may appear confusing at first glance, this brief overview should help you separate the wheat from the chaff.

Before we begin, I'd like to say a few words about self-diagnosis and treatment. As a rule, I tell patients that it's safe to experiment with an herbal remedy for a mild complaint, such as a runny nose or an upset stomach. However, self-diagnosis based on symptoms (complaints) can be risky business. Therefore, if the symptoms are severe, if they get worse despite simple measures, or if the symptoms linger for more than a few days, see a doctor.

DIFFERENCES BETWEEN HERBAL AND PRESCRIPTION MEDICATION

Although drugs can trace their roots to herbs, there are fundamental differences between the two branches of the family. For instance, herbal remedies are significantly less expensive than prescription medication. They're also less likely to cause side effects—and if they do, the side effects are usually mild and disappear once the herb is stopped. That's because herbal therapies work differently than do prescription drugs: Herbs can take as long as four to six weeks to reach peak effectiveness, whereas prescription drugs work within minutes (however, potent drugs can also cause side effects just as quickly). Although herbs are generally safe, they can interact with prescription medication. *Therefore, if you take prescription medication, check with your physician before taking an herbal supplement.*

HOW TO TELL IF AN HERB IS "WORKING"

Herbs contain hundreds, even thousands, of ingredients that work together to promote health by supporting the body's own healing abilities.
As a result, herbs have a subtle effect on the body that is often difficult to
measure. Nevertheless, if symptoms remain unchanged after taking an
herb for two to four weeks, or if there is any doubt, stop taking the herb
and see if the symptoms recur. Bear in mind, though, that a lack of improvement may not be the herb's fault. The blame can often be traced to
an inferior herbal product (which was bought because it's cheaper), failure
to take the herb as directed, an improper diagnosis, or choosing the wrong
herb in the first place. Which leads us to the next topic.

HOW TO SELECT A QUALITY HERBAL PRODUCT

Dr. Andrew Weil, a noted authority on herbal medicine, suggests the following guidelines:

- **Become knowledgeable by doing your homework.** For instance, read a reputable book on herbs, talk with your doctor,
  consult a medical herbalist (experts in herbal medicine; contact
  The American Herbalists Guild [see the Resources section on
  page 177] to find one in your area). Watchdog organizations
  also provide information about nutritional and herbal supplements *(www.consumerlabs.com)*.
- **Select the most effective form by choosing a *standardized*
  herbal product if one is available.** Standardized products are
  assayed (checked in a laboratory) to make sure that they contain a specified amount of a particular ingredient. However, be
  advised that standardization doesn't guarantee potency or
  quality. A product is only as good as the raw ingredients and
  the quality of the manufacturing process. Bulk herbs that are
  stored in open bins quickly lose their potency, and powdered
  herbs are subject to *adulteration* (addition of a substance other
  than the desired herb). Although adulterants usually consist of

the wrong part of the plant or the wrong herb, they can also include heavy metals such as mercury and lead, toxic pesticides, and bacterial or fungal contaminants. With regard to cost, liquid and solid herbal extracts offer the best buy for the money. Finally, it's generally better to select a product that contains a single herb, instead of one that tries to cover all the bases with a shopping list of herbal ingredients. Herbalists, however, can get away with mixing and matching herbs, since they know which ones work best together.

• **Buy from reputable companies.** I recommend purchasing herbs from companies that have an established reputation (not to be confused with companies that advertise the most). Select a company that adheres to "good manufacturing practices" (see page 161). Companies that I trust include all the companies listed on page 162, plus the Eclectic Institute, Herbalist & Alchemist, Inc., and GAIA Herbs, Inc.

HOW TO READ AN HERBAL SUPPLEMENT LABEL

The following information is typically listed on an herbal supplement label (See the chart on page 166). Items in bold type are discussed in further detail.

Supplement Facts

Serving Size: *two 160 mg softgels*

Amount per serving *(two softgels)*	% **DV***
Saw palmetto *(Serenoa repens)* **Extract (10:1):**	320 mg
Extracted from **saw palmetto berries**	
Standardized to yield **85–95% fatty acids and sterols**	
Other ingredients: gelatin, glycerine, and water	

Saw palmetto **helps maintain proper urine flow**[†]

Usage: Take two softgels daily or as directed by your qualified health consultant.

*Daily Value: Not Established

[†]*This statement has not been authorized by the Food and Drug Administration. This product is not intended to diagnose, treat, cure, or prevent any disease.*

Here's a translation of the label:

- **Serving size** specifies the number of capsules that must be taken to yield the recommended daily amount.
- **Saw palmetto** *(Serenoa repens):* Herbs are identified by a common name, which comes first (saw palmetto), followed by a botanical name that is enclosed in parentheses and italicized *(Serenoa repens)*. The part of the herb that was used to make the formulation **(saw palmetto berries)** is also identified.
- **Extract:** A solvent, usually water or alcohol, is used to "extract" (withdraw) an herb's active ingredients. Water extracts

water-soluble ingredients, whereas alcohol extracts fat-soluble items such as fatty acids, sterols, and other substances that are water-insoluble. Extracts are categorized by the concentration of herb relative to the amount of solvent. *Herbal infusions* (a fancy name for tea) and *tinctures* contain more solvent than herb, while the reverse is true for *liquid* and *solid* extracts. Most popular herbal *liquid tinctures* contain one part herb to five or ten parts solvent (written as 1:5 or 1:10 herbal tincture). An herbal *liquid extract* contains at least the same amount or more herbal product than solvent. For instance, a 2:1 liquid extract contains two parts herb for every part solvent. Finally, an herbal *solid extract* usually contains at least four parts herb for every part solvent (expressed as 4:1 solid extract)—or, in this case, ten parts herb to one part solvent **(10:1).**

- **Standardization:** Whenever the active ingredient is known, it's possible to *standardize* a product that contains a specified percentage of *active ingredient*(s)—for instance, **85–95% fatty acids and sterols.** An *active ingredient* is the chemical that presumably accounts for an herb's healing properties. Products can also be standardized to contain a certain concentration of herbal ingredients—for example, a standardized 10:1 herbal extract.

- **Other ingredients:** Anything that is contained in the product other than the pure herb should be listed in this section. Unless stated otherwise, **gelatin** vitamin capsules are derived from processed animal collagen (for instance, animal hoofs). "Vegicaps," on the other hand, are made from vegetable protein and **glycerine** (a fat derivative).

- **Daily value:** Unlike vitamins and minerals, herbs don't have a recommended daily value (amount).

- **Structure/function statement:** The Food and Drug Administration permits manufacturers to describe how an herb affects the body's structure or function—for example, they can state that saw palmetto **"helps maintain proper urine flow"** — as long as they also include the disclaimer listed above denoted by an asterisk (†).

- **Usage:** The recommended dosage may vary depending on a
person's weight, medical condition, other medications, and the
nature of the condition being treated. For instance, if a man
weighs over 200 pounds, I recommend taking three instead of
two 160 mg saw palmetto softgels daily.

Note: Liquid herbal preparations are measured in "cc" (cubic centimeter)
or "ml" (milliliter) amounts (the two measurements are equivalent). Common liquid measurements include the following: One teaspoon equals
5 ccs, one tablespoon equals 15 ccs, and one ounce equals 30 ccs. Liquid
herbal tinctures or extracts are also dispensed by the drop (one dropperful
equals approximately forty drops).

Dried herbs are dispensed by weight. One heaping teaspoon of dried
herb averages between one and four and a half grams (flowers average one
gram, bark averages four and a half grams, and the remaining herbal
parts weigh somewhere in between).

Notes

CHAPTER 2

[1]Jeffrey P. Weiss and Jerry G. Blaivas, "A Practical Approach to Nocturia in Adults," *Contemporary Urology* 10 (8) (1998): 15–19.

[2]Michael J. Barry et al., "The Natural History of Patients with Benign Prostatic Hyperplasia as Diagnosed by North American Urologists," *Journal of Urology* 157 (January 1997): 10–15.

[3]Joseph E. Osterling, "Benign Prostatic Hyperplasia: Medical and Minimally Invasive Treatment Options," *New England Journal of Medicine* 352 (2) (January 12, 1995): 106.

[4]Cheryl Guttman, "Finasteride's Effect on Men without BPH Studied," *Urology Times* 28 (August 2000): 10–11.

[5]Kevin T. McVary, "Prostatic Disease: Options and Advances," *Audio-Digest Urology* 22 (12) (1999): 1.

[6]Franklin C. Lowe and James C. Ku, "Phytotherapy in Treatment of Benign Prostatic Hyperplasia: A Critical Review," *Urology* 48 (1) (1996): 12.

[7]S. K. Clinton and W. J. Visek, "Wheat Bran and the Induction of Intestinal Bezo(a)pyrene Hydroxylase by Dietary Benzo(a)pyrene," *Journal of Nutrition* 119 (3) (1989): 395–402.

[8]Elizabeth A. Platz, et al., "Physical Activity and Benign Prostatic Hyperplasia," *Archives of Internal Medicine* 158 (November 23, 1998): 2349–2356.

[9]J. Koskimäki, et al., "Association of Smoking with Lower Urinary Tract Symptoms," *Journal of Urology* 159 (May 1998) 1580–1582.

[10]Timothy J. Wilt, "Saw Palmetto Extracts for Treatment of Benign Prostatic Hyperplasia: A Systematic Review," *Journal of the American Medical Association* 280 (18) (November 11, 1996): 1604–1609.

[11]Russell H. Greenfield, "*Pygeum africanum* for the Treatment of Mild-to-Moderate Benign Prostatic Hyperplasia," *Alternative Medicine Alert* 2 (2) (1999): 14.

[12]Glenn S. Gerber, "Phytotherapy in the Treatment of Benign Prostatic Hyperplasia," in Culley C. Carson, ed., *Mediguide to Urology* (New York: Lawrence DellaCorte Publications, Inc., 1998), pp. 1–7.

[13]E. W. Rugendorff et al., "Results of Treatment with Pollen Extract (Cernilton N) in Chronic Prostatitis and Prostodynia," *British Journal of Urology* 71 (1993): 433–438.

[14]Rocio Paola Yaffar, ed., "BPH, The Other Side of the Coin," *Life Extension Magazine* (February 1999): 13–15.

CHAPTER 3

[1]Angelo M. DeMarzo, Donald S. Coffey, and William G. Nelson, "New Concepts in Tissue Specificity for Prostate Cancer and Benign Prostatic Hyperplasia," *Urology* 53 (Supplement 3A) (March 1999): 35.

[2]Bradley R. Hennenfent, *The Prostatitis Syndromes* (Smithshire, IL: The Prostatitis Foundation, 1996), pp. 1–97.

[3]Julia Talsma, "NIH-Backed Event Formalizes Approach to Syndrome," *Urology Times* 28 (4) (2000): 32.

[4]Ibid., 32–33.

[5]J. Curtis Nickel and Ron Sorensen, "Transurethral Microwave Therapy For Nonbacterial Prostatitis: A Randomized Double-Blind Sham Controlled Study Using New Prostatitis Specific Assessment Questionnaires," *The Journal of Urology* 155 (June 1996) 1950–1955.

[6]H. M. Drane et al., "The Chance Discovery of Oestrogenic Activity in Laboratory Rat Cake," *Food Cosmetology and Toxicology* 13 (1975): 491–492.

[7]Alan R. Gaby, "Allergy Elimination Diet 'A'," Nutritional Therapy in Medical Practice Conference, Seattle, Washington, October 25–28, 1996.

[8]Glenn S. Gerber, "Phytotherapy in the Treatment of Benign Prostatic Hyperplasia," Culley C. Carson, ed. *Mediguide to Urology* (New York: Lawrence DellaCorte Publications, Inc., 1998), pp. 1–8.

[9]E. W. Rugendorff et al., "Results of Treatment with Pollen Extract (Cernilton N) in Chronic Prostatitis and Prostodynia," *British Journal of Urology* 71 (1993): 433–438.

[10]Rosebud O. Roberts et al, "Prevalence of a Physician-Assigned Diagnosis of Prostatitis: The Olmsted County Study of Urinary Symptoms and Health Status Among Men," *Urology* 51(4) (1998): 578.

[11]Michael T. Murray, "Echinacea: Pharmacology and Clinical Applications," *American Journal of Natural Medicine* 2 (1) (January/February 1995): 18–24.

[12]Michael T. Murray, *The Healing Power of Herbs,* 2d ed. (Rocklin, CA: Prima Publishing, 1995), p. 215.

[13]David Winston, *Herbal Therapeutics: Specific Indications For Herbs & Herbal Formulas*, 5th ed. (Broadway, NJ: Herbalist Therapeutics Research Library, 1996), p. 38.

[14]Joel L. Marmar et al., "Semen Zinc Levels in Infertile and Post Vasectomy Patients and Patients with Prostatitis," *Fertility and Sterility* 26 (11) (1975): 1057–1063.

[15]Jonathan V. Wright, "D-Mannose and Infection," in *Dr. Jonathan V. Wright's Nutrition & Healing* (Phoenix: Nutrition & Healing, Inc., June 1999): 1,6.

[16]Daniel A. Shoskes et al., "Quercetin in Men with Category III Chronic Prostatitis: A Preliminary Prospective, Double-Blind, Placebo-Controlled Trial," *Urology* 54 (6) (1999): 960–963.

[17]Joseph E. Pizzorno, Jr. and Michael T. Murray, *Textbook of Natural Medicine*, 2d Ed. (NY: Churchill Livingston, 1999), p. 895.

[18]Y. Aso et al., "Preventive Effect of Lactobacillus Casei Preparation on the Recurrence of Superficial Bladder Cancer in a Double-Blind Trial," *European Urology* 27 (1995): 104–109.

[19]Jeffrey S. Bland and Sara H. Benum, *Genetic Nutritioneering: How You Can Modify Inherited Traits and Live a Longer, Healthier Life* (Los Angeles: Keats Publishing, 1999), pp. 133–134.

[20]Mark W. Litwin et al., "The National Institutes of Health Chronic Prostatitis Symptom Index: Development and Validation of a New Outcome Measure," *Journal of Urology* 162 (August 1999): 374.

CHAPTER 4

[1]William R. Fair, "Diet and Lifestyle Changes," *Audio-Digest Urology* 24 (1) (2001): 1.

[2]June M. Chan et al., "Plasma Insulin-Like Growth Factor-1 and Prostate Cancer Risk: A Prospective Study," *Science* 279 (January 23, 1998): 563–566.

[3]Richard R. Kerr, editor-in-chief, "In Brief," *Urology Times* 28 (8) (2000): 3.

[4]E. Bernal-Delgado et al., "The Association Between Vasectomy and Prostate Cancer: A Systematic Review of the Literature," *Fertility and Sterility* 70 (1998): 191–200.

[5]J. E. Oesterling et al., "Serum Prostate-Specific Antigen in a Community-Based Population of Healthy Men: Establishment of Age-Specific Reference Ranges," *Journal of the American Medical Association* 270 (1993): 860.

[6]Alan W. Partin and Ray E. Stutzman, "Elevated Prostate-Specific Antigen, Abnormal Prostate Evaluation on Digital Rectal Exam, and Transrectal Ultrasound and Prostate Biopsy," *Urologic Clinics of North America* 25 (4) (1998): 583.

[7]Patrick C. Walsh et al., "Cancer Control and Quality of Life Following Anatomical Radical Retropubic Prostatectomy: Results at 10 Years," *Journal of Urology* 152 (1994): 1831.

[8]David J. Brenner et al., "Second Malignancies in Prostate Carcinoma Patients after Radiotherapy Compared with Surgery," *Cancer* 88 (2) (January 15, 2000): 398–406.

[9]Charles E. Myers, "Radiation Therapy: Are You Cured?" *Prostate Forum Newsletter* 5 (9) (March 2000): 2.

[10]E. Ernst and B. R. Cassileth, "The Prevalence of Complementary/Alternative Medicine in Cancer," *Cancer* 83 (4) (August 15, 1998): 777–782.

[11]Michael Lerner, *Choices in Healing* (Cambridge, MA: MIT Press, 1996), p. 111.

[12]H. Schipper, C. R. Goh, T. L. Wang, "Shifting the Cancer Paradigm: Must We Kill to Cure?" *Journal of Clinical Oncology* 13 (4) (April, 1995): 801.

[13]Jeffrey S. Bland et al., *Clinical Nutrition: A Functional Approach* (Gig Harbor: WA: The Institute for Functional Medicine, 1999), p. 78.

[14]Edward Giovannucci et al., "Intake of Carotenoids and Retinol in Relation to Risk of Prostate Cancer," *Journal of the National Cancer Institute* 87 (1995): 1767–1776.

[15]J. P. Carter et al., "Hypothesis: Dietary Management May Improve Survival from Nutritionally Linked Cancers Based on Analysis of Representative Cases," *Journal of the American College of Nutrition* 12 (1993): 209–226.

[16]Olli P. Heinonen et al., "Prostate Cancer and Supplementation with Alpha-tocopherol and Beta-carotene: Incidence and Mortality in a Controlled Trial," *Journal of the National Cancer Institute* 90 (6) (1998): 440–446.

[17]N. R. Cook et al., "ß–Carotene Supplementation for Patients with Low Baseline Levels and Decreased Risks of Total and Prostate Carcinoma," *Cancer* 86 (November 1, 1999): 1783–1792.

[18]Shutsung Liao et al., "Growth Inhibition and Regression of Human Prostate and Breast Tumors in Athymic Mice by Tea Epigallocatechin Gallate," *Cancer Letters* 96 (1995): 239–243.

[19]Xiaolin Zi et al., "A Flavonoid Antioxidant, Silymarin, Inhibits Activation of erbB1 Signaling and Induces Cyclin-dependent Kinase Inhibitors, G1 Arrest, and Anticarcinogenic Effects in Human Prostate Carcinoma DU145 Cells," *Cancer Research* 58 (9) (1998): 1920–1929.

[20]Joe Bina and B. R. Lokesh, "Effect of Curcumin and Capsaicin on Arachidonic Acid Metabolism and Lysomal Enzyme Secretion by Rat Peritoneal Macrophages," *Lipids* 32 (11) (1997): 1173–1179.

[21]Kerry Bone, "The Story of Boswellia," *Nutrition & Healing* 6 (4) (April 1999): 3–4

[22]Myers, *Prostate Forum* 3 (12) (December 1999): 7.

[23]Myers, *Prostate Forum* 5 (7) (July 2000): pp. 4–5.

[24]John T. Pinto et al., "Effects of Garlic Thioallyl Derivitates on Growth, Glutathione Concentration, and Polyamine Formation of Human Prostate Carcinoma Cells in Culture," *American Journal of Clinical Nutrition* 66 (1997): 398–405.

[25]Eric J. Small et al., "Prospective Trial of the Herbal Supplement PC-SPES in Patients with Progressive Prostate Cancer," *Journal of Clinical Oncology* 18 (21) (November 1, 2000): 3595–3602.

[26]Thomas M. Burton, "In Trials, Potion of Herbs Slows Prostate Cancer," *Wall Street Journal* 17 May 2000, B1.

[27]Larry C. Clark et al., "Effects of Selenium Supplementation for Cancer Prevention in Patients with Carcinoma of the Skin," *Journal of the American Medical Association* 276 (24) (December 25, 1996): 1957–1963.

[28]P. J. du Toit et al., "The Effects of Essential Fatty Acids on Growth and Urokinase-type Plasminogen Activator Production in Human Prostate DU145 Cells," *Prostaglandins Leukotrienes Essential Fatty Acids*, 55 (1996): 173–177.

[29]Myers, *Prostate Forum* 5 (7) (July 2000): p. 2.

[30]J. Liang, "Inhibitory effect of zinc on human prostatic carcinoma cell growth," *Prostate* 1999, 40: 200–207.

[31]Paolo Lissoni et al., "Reversal of Clinical Resistance to LHRH Analogue in Metastatic Prostate Cancer by the Pineal Hormone Melatonin: Efficacy of LHRH Analogue Plus Melatonin in Patients on LHRH Analogue Alone," *European Urology* 31 (1997): 178–181.

[32]K. J. Pienta et al., "Inhibition of Spontaneous Metastasis in a Rat Prostate Cancer Model by Oral Administration of Modified Citrus Pectin," *Journal of the National Cancer Institute* 87 (1995): 348–353.

[33]Myers, *Prostate Forum Newsletter* 4 (9) (September 1999): 1–3.

[34]Ibid., 4(6) (June 1999): 6–7.

[35]David W. Lamson and Matthew S. Brignall, "Antioxidants and Cancer Therapy II: Quick Reference Guide," *Alternative Medicine Review* 5 (2) (2000): 152–163.

[36]Ibid., 4 (8) (August 1999): 6–7.

[37]E. J. Lien, "The Use of Chinese Herbal Medicine in Cancer Prevention and Chemotherapy: A Survey," *Oriental Healing Arts Bulletin* 13 (1988): 59–68

[38]Hiroaki Nanba, "Maitake D-fraction: Healing and Preventive Potential for Cancer," *Journal of Orthomolecular Medicine* 12 (1) (1997): 43–49.

[39]Kenneth Jones, "Reishi Mushroom, Ancient Medicine in Modern Times," *Alternative & Complementary Therapies* 4 (4) (August 1998): 256–266.

[40]H. Yarbro et al., "N-acetylcysteine: A Significant Chemoprotective Adjuvant," *Seminars on Oncology* 1 (Suppl) (1983): 1.

[41]S. Klimberg, "Prevention of Radiogenic Side Effects Using Glutamine-Enriched Elemental Diets," *Recent Results in Cancer Research* 121 (1991): 283–285.

[42]Y. Mao et al., "Pectin-supplemented Enteral Diet Reduces the Severity of Methtrexate Induced Enterocolitis in Rats," *Scandanavian Journal of Gastroenterology* 31 (6) (1996): 558–567

[43]S. W. Ha, "Enhancement of Radiation Response of C3H Mouse Fsa II Tumor by Extract of Ginkgo biloba (Meeting Abstract)," International Congress of Radiation Oncology 1993, June 21–25, 1993, Kyoto, Japan, 268.

[44]Lamson, *Alternative Medicine Review* 5 (2) (2000): 154.

[45]Lerner, *Choices in Healing,* p. 384.

[46]P. M. Kidd, "The Use of Mushroom Glycans and Proteoglycans in Cancer Treatment," *Alternative Medicine Review* 5 (2000): 4–27.

[47]Donald L. Lamm et al., "Megadose Vitamins in Bladder Cancer: A Double-blind Clinical Trial," *Journal of Urology* 151 (January 1994): 21–26.

[48]D. S. Michaud et al., "Fluid Intake and the Risk of Bladder Cancer in Men," *New England Journal of Medicine* 340 (May 6, 1999): 1390–1397.

[49]Lester A. Mitscher and Victoria Dolby, *The Green Tea Book* (Garden City Park, NY: Avery Publishing Group, 1998), p. 76.

[50]Y. Aso et al., "Preventive Effect of *Lactobacillus Casei* Preparation on the Recurrence of Superficial Bladder Cancer in a Double-Blind Trial," *European Urology* 27 (1995): 104–109.

[51]Burton M. Berkson, "A Triple Antioxidant Approach to the Treatment of Hepatitis C Using Alpha-Lipoic (Thioctic Acid) Silymarin, Selenium, and Other Fundamental Neutraceuticals," *Clinical Practice of Alternative Medicine* 1 (1) (Spring 2000): 27–33.

[52]Dean Shrock, Raymond F. Palmer, and Bonnie Taylor, "Effects of a Psychosocial Intervention on Survival Among Patients with Stage 1 Breast and Prostate Cancer: A Matched Case-Control Study," *Alternative Therapies* 5 (3) (1999): 49–55.

Resources

ALTERNATIVE CANCER THERAPIES

Books
- John Boik, *Cancer & Natural Medicine: A Textbook of Basic Science and Clinical Research* (Princeton, MN: Oregon Medical Press, 1995).
- Burton Goldberg, *Definitive Guide to Cancer* (Fife, WA: Future Medicine Publishing, Inc., 1997).
- Michael Lerner, *Choices in Healing* (Cambridge, MA: MIT Press, 1994).
- Ralph W. Moss, *Herbs Against Cancer* (Brooklyn, NY: Equinox Press, 1998).
- Kedar N. Prasad, *Vitamins in Cancer Prevention and Treatment* (Rochester, VT: Healing Arts Press, 1994).
- Charles B. Simone, *Cancer & Nutrition* (Garden City Park, NY: Avery Publishing Group, Inc., 1994).

Internet Websites
- FDA Guide to Choosing Medical Treatments: http://www.fda.gov//oashi/aids/fdaguide.html
- Internet Resources on Cancer: http://cpmcnet.columbia.edu/dept/rosenthal/Guide6.html
- National Center for Complementary and Alternative Medicine: http://nccam.nih.gov

ALTERNATIVE MEDICINE

Organizations

- American College of Advancement in Medicine, 23121 Verdugo Drive, Suite 204, Laguna Hills, CA 92653; (800) 532-3688; website: http://www.acam.org
- American Holistic Medical Society, 6728 Old McLean Village Drive, McLean, VA 22101-3906; (703) 556-9245; website: www.holisticmedicine.org
- National Center for Complementary and Alternative Medicine Clearing House, P.O. Box 8218, Silver Spring, MD 20907-8218; (888) 644-6226; website: http://nccam.nih.gov

Books

- Elliott S. Dacher, *Whole Healing* (NewYork: Penguin Books, 1996).
- Leo Galland, *Power Healing* (NewYork: Random House, 1997).
- Burton Goldberg, *Alternative Medicine* (Fife, WA: Future Medicine Publishing, Inc., 1994).
- James S. Gordon, *Manifesto for a New Medicine* (NewYork: Addison-Wesley Publishing, Inc., 1996).
- Michael T. Murray and Joseph E. Pizzorno, Jr., *Textbook of Natural Medicine*, 2nd ed. (NewYork: Churchill Livingston, 1999).
- Andrew Weil, *Natural Health, Natural Medicine* (Boston: Houghton Mifflin Co., 1998).

Newsletters

- *Dr. Andrew Weil's Self-Healing,* Thorne Communications, Inc., 42 Pleasant St., Watertown, MA 02172; (617) 926-0200.
- *Alternative Medicine Alert,* American Health Consultants; (800) 688-2421.

BIOFEEDBACK

Organization
- Association for Applied Psychophysiology and Biofeedback, 10200 West 44th Avenue, Suite 304, Wheat Ridge, CO 80033; website: http://www.aapb.org

GUIDED IMAGERY

Organization
- The Academy for Guided Imagery, P.O. Box 2070, Mill Valley, CA 94942; (800) 726-2070; website: http://www. interactiveimagery.com/

Book
- Martin L. Rossman, *Healing Yourself: A Step-by-Step Program for Better Health Through Imagery* (New York: Pocket Books, 1989).

HERBAL MEDICINE

Organizations
- American Botanical Council, P.O. Box 144345, Austin, TX; (512) 926-4900; website: http://www.herbalgram.com
- The American Herbalists Guild, 1931 Gaddis Road, Canton, GA 30115; (770) 751-6021; website: http://www.american herbalistsguild.com

Books and Journals
- James A. Duke, *The Green Pharmacy* (Emmaus, PA: Rodale Press, 1997).

- Joe Graedon and Teresa Graedon, *The People's Pharmacy Guide to Home and Herbal Remedies* (New York: St. Martin's Press, 1999).
- *HerbalGram,* American Botanical Council, P.O. Box 201660, Austin, TX 78720; (512) 331-8868. Published quarterly.
- J. M. Jellin, F. Batz, and K. Hitchens, *Pharmacist's Letter/ Prescriber's Letter Natural Medicines Comprehensive Database* (Stockton, CA: Therapeutic Research Facility, 2001).
- *PDR for Herbal Medicines* (Montvale, NJ: Medical Economics Co., 2000).
- Michael T. Murray, *The Healing Power of Herbs* (Rocklin, CA: Prima Publishing, 1995).
- Varro E. Tyler, *Herbs of Choice: The Therapeutic Use of Phytomedicinals* (Binghamton, NY: Pharmaceutical Products Press, Inc., 1994).

Internet Websites

- Joe Graedon and Teresa Graedon, The People's Pharmacy: http://www.peoplespharmacy.com
- Phytochemical and Ethnobotanical Databases: http://www. ars-grin.gov/duke/
- U.S. Pharmacopoeia: http://www.usp.org

MACROBIOTICS

Books

- Michio Kushi, *The Macrobiotic Way* (Garden City, NY: Avery Publishing Group, 1993).
- Michio Kushi and Aveline Kushi, *Macrobiotic Diet* (Tokyo: Japan Publishers, Inc., 1993).

Internet Website

- Macrobiotics Online: http://www.macrobiotics.org/

NUTRITIONAL SUPPLEMENTS

Books
- Michael T. Murray, *Encyclopedia of Nutritional Supplements* (Rocklin, CA: Prima Publishing, 1996).
- Michael T. Murray, *Natural Alternatives to Over-the-Counter and Prescription Drugs* (New York: William Morrow & Co., 1994).

Internet Website
- U.S. Pharmacopoeia: http://www.usp.org

ORGANIC FOOD

Books
- Jeanne Heifetz, *Green Groceries—A Mail Order Guide to Organic Foods* (New York: HarperPerennial, 1992).
- *Rodale's All-New Encyclopedia of Organic Gardening* (Emmaus, PA: Rodale, 1992).

Mail-Order Resources
- Diamond Organics (800) 922-2396.
- Goldmine National Foods (800) 475-3663.

TRADITIONAL CHINESE MEDICINE

Organization
- American Association of Oriental Medicine, 433 Front Street, Catasauqua, PA 18032; (610) 266-1433.

Books
- Harriett Beinfield and Efrem Korngold, *Between Heaven and Earth* (New York: Ballantine Books, 1991).

- Ted J. Kaptchuk, *The Web That Has No Weaver: Understanding Chinese Medicine* (Chicago: Contemporary Publishing Group, Inc., 2000).

Internet Website

- National Certification Commission for Acupuncture and Oriental Medicine: http://www.nccaom.org

UROLOGY

Organizations

- American Foundation for Urologic Disease (AFUD), 300 W. Pratt St., Suite 401, Baltimore, MD 21201; (800) 242-2383; website: http://www.afud.org/
- American Urological Association, Inc., 1120 N. Charles Street, Baltimore, MD 21201-5559; (410) 727-1100; website: http://www.auanet.org
- CaP Cure, 1250 Fourth Street, Suite 360, Santa Monica, CA 90401; (310) 458-2873; website: http://www.capcure.org
- The Interstitial Cystitis Association, 51 Monroe Street, Suite 1402, Rockville, MD 20850; (800) help.ica; website: http://www.ichelp.com
- National Association for Continence, P.O. Box 8310, Spartanburg, SC 29305; (800) Bladder; website: www.nafc.org
- Patients Advocates for Advanced Cancer Treatments (PAACT), P.O. Box 141695, Grand Rapids, MI 49514-1695; (616) 453-1477; website: http://www.paactusa.org/
- Prostate Cancer Research Institute, 5777 W. Century Boulevard, Suite 885, Los Angeles, CA 90045; (310) 743-2116; website: http://www.prostate-cancer.org
- US-TOO Prostate Cancer Survivor Support Groups, 930 N. York Rd., Suite 50, Hinsdale, IL 60521-2993; (630) 323-1002; website: http://www.ustoo.com

Books and Booklets

- Barry McCarthy and Emily McCarthy, *Male Sexual Awareness* (New York: Carroll & Graf Publishers, Inc., 1998).
- Charles E. "Snuffy" Myers, Jr., Sara Sgarlat Steck, and Rose Sgarlat Myers, *Eating Your Way to Better Health* (Charlottesville, VA: Rivanna Health Publications, Inc., 2000).
- J. C. Nickel, ed., *Textbook of Prostatitis* (Herndon, VA: Isis Medical Media, 2000).
- *Nutrition & Prostate Cancer: A Monograph from the CaP CURE Nutrition Project,* CaP Cure, 1250 Fourth Street, Suite 360, Santa Monica, CA 90401; (310) 458-2873.
- Robert H. Phillips, *Coping with Prostate Cancer* (Garden City Park, NY: Avery Publishing Group, 1994).
- *Prostate Cancer and Bone Metastases,* CaP Cure, 1250 Fourth Street, Suite 360, Santa Monica, CA 90401; (310) 458-2873.
- *Prostate Cancer Resource Guide,* American Foundation for Urologic Disease (AFUD), 300 W. Pratt St., Suite 401, Baltimore, MD 21201; (800) 242-2383.
- Grannum Sant, *Interstitial Cystitis* (New York: Lippincott-Raven, 1997).

Internet Websites

- CancerNet: http://cancernet.nci.nih.gov/
- Gary Huckabay's *Prostate Pointers:* http://www.prostate pointers.org/
- Prostate Forum: http://www.prostateforum.com/
- University of Pennsylvania: http://www.oncolink.upenn.edu/

Newsletters

- *Cancer Communications Newsletter,* Patients Advocates for Advanced Cancer Treatments (PAACT), P.O. Box 141695, Grand Rapids, MI 49514-1695; (616) 453-1477.
- *PCRInsights,* Prostate Cancer Research Institute, 5777 W. Century Boulevard, Suite 885, Los Angeles, CA 90045; (310) 743-2116.

- *Prostate Forum*, P.O. Box 6696, Charlotttesville, VA 22906; (800) 305-2432.
- *US TOO Prostate Cancer Communicator,* US-TOO Prostate Cancer Survivor Support Groups, 930 N. York Road, Suite 50, Hinsdale, IL 60521-2993; (630) 323-1002.

YOGA

Organization
- International Association of Yoga Therapists, P.O. Box 1386, Locuer Lake, CA 951457; (707) 928-9898; website: http://www.yrec.org

Books
- Georg Feuerstein and Larry Payne, *Yoga for Dummies* (New York: IDG Books Worldwide, Inc., 1999).
- B. K. S. Iyengar, *Light on Yoga* (New York: Schocken Books, 1979).
- Swami Vishnudevananda, *The Complete Illustrated Book of Yoga* (New York: Harmony Books, 1980).

Index

About the Author

After graduating from Indiana University School of Medicine, Mark W. McClure, M.D., received his urology training at the University of Pennsylvania. Since starting practice in 1981, he has appeared on radio and television, written numerous articles and several textbook chapters, and lectured extensively on various aspects of complementary medicine. Since 1996, he has served as medical editor for *Health & Healing,* a Research Triangle–based health newspaper. In 1997, Dr. McClure founded Landmark Urology and Complementary Medicine—one of the first urology practices in the United States to offer both conventional and complementary medicine. He is board certified in both urology and holistic medicine and currently practices urology and complementary medicine in Raleigh, North Carolina.

Dr. McClure is donating half of his net proceeds from the sale of *Smart Medicine for a Healthy Prostate* to prostate cancer research and other charitable organizations. He encourages others to donate generously to prostate cancer research and patient education.